P9-CDD-862

METRICS

Ch 3 & 4: how to encavage heath behaviors
without tempting ppl to
skew statistics?

millenium development goals
→ who decides these issues
are most pressing?

logistics of collecting data
— malaria treatments

catch-22 of needing data
but not predetermind indicators
(p. 120)

CRITICAL GLOBAL HEALTH · *Evidence, Efficacy, Ethnography*
A series edited by Vincanne Adams and João Biehl

METRICS What Counts in Global Health

VINCANNE ADAMS, EDITOR Duke University Press · Durham London · 2016

Ch 1 & 2: loss of human aspect, reduction of
cultural, ethnographic differences (p. 41)
- interface of capitalism & 12
medecine (p. 37, 38)

Q: What is DALY & QALY?
- importance of stories

- importance of assumptions
in metrics

Critique: critical of metrics, but without
evidence to back it up?

- numbers taken at face value

THIS BOOK IS DEDICATED TO
MY MENTOR, TEACHER, AND FRIEND,
RONNIE FRANKENBERG.

© 2016 DUKE UNIVERSITY PRESS. All rights reserved.
Printed in the United States of America on acid-free paper ∞
Designed by Courtney Leigh Baker and typeset in Trade Gothic
and Arno by Tseng Information Systems, Inc.

Library of Congress Cataloging-in-Publication Data
Metrics : what counts in global health / Vincanne Adams, editor
pages cm — (Critical global health)
Includes bibliographical references and index.
ISBN 978-0-8223-6083-4 (hardcover : alk. paper)
ISBN 978-0-8223-6097-1 (pbk. : alk. paper)
ISBN 978-0-8223-7448-0 (e-book)
1. World health—Research. 2. World health—Econometric models.
3. Health status indicators—Evaluation. 4. Social indicators—
Evaluation. I. Adams, Vincanne, 1959– editor. II. Series: Critical
global health.
RA441.M48 2016
362.1072—dc23
2015033349

Cover art: Tara Donovan, Colony, 2004 (detail). Pencils. 7.6 × 337.8 ×
198.1 cm. Photograph by Tom Barratt, courtesy of Pace Gallery.
© Tara Donovan, courtesy of Pace Gallery.

CONTENTS

INTRODUCTION VINCANNE ADAMS

The shift from *international health development* to *global health* in the sixty-year-old postcolonial infrastructure of transnational health aid is not a simple case of new bottles for old wine. Emergent trends attending to the desires for global health reveal complex transformations in the practices of audit, funding, and intervention. One of the most important features of this shift has been the growing push for and reliance upon specific kinds of quantitative metrics that make use of evidence-based statistical measures, experimental research platforms, and cost-effectiveness rubrics for even the most intractable health problems and most promising interventions. Anthropologists have been writing in interesting ways about these shifts, and we sense a need for both applause and caution in the embrace of these rubrics for doing health work in global ways. This book offers a series of ethnographic explorations of these trends, focusing on the on-the-ground realities of what we might call *metrics work* while also investigating the expectations and accomplishments that the *metrics* create, for better or worse, in global health today.

Global Health: Rupture and Persistence

The phrase *global health* is used to name a variety of familiar and unfamiliar activities, most of which are in perpetual motion. Chapter 1 offers a more complete overview of the central argument of the book, mapping the trajectories metrics have taken in the conceptualization of global health and serving as a longer orienting chapter for the collection. Here it is useful to note that in this volume we see global health as *both* a response to exigencies of finance, data, and outcomes that have defined the postwar world of international health *and* a utopian proposition to escape, if not transcend, the problems and perceived lack of success of these arrangements and exigencies. The links among economy, sovereignty, and the politics of knowledge that have shaped the use of metrics over the past decades in this field suggest that global health strives toward forms of knowledge that are distinguished from those found in an era of postwar, postcolonial international health. It is worth noting at the outset that this claim invites scrutiny from a number of positions and empirical grounds.

Recall, for instance, that postwar international health was, in its own way, a response to what came before it: colonial health and the demands of empire that such health was attendant upon. How global health might be seen as rupture rather than continuity and the specific resemblances it has to earlier forms of health aid in *both* the colonial and postcolonial eras is perhaps most visible not just in the efforts to count things but in how counting things has worked in relation to other political and economic institutions.

For instance, global health is not the first to think "globally." Colonial tropical medicine configured the global in its own ways. Similarly postwar international health efforts imagined a worldly set of impacts and interventions. There are differences, however, in how these eras imagined their geographic reach and how they undertook to count health, especially in relation to economics. These differences help us distinguish what is new and what is old in today's global health metrics.

Colonial tropical disease maps of the spread of yellow fever, dengue, tuberculosis, and smallpox, and the mapping sciences deployed to measure these, were crafted under the assumption that the reach of empire went beyond sovereign borders (Anderson 2006; Tilley 2011). Colonial health efforts not only imagined geographic continuities across continents and oceans but also across racial, ethnic, and national territories, and intervention and mapping projects counted in ways that authorized and ensured the expansion and stability of these empires (Birn et al. 2009; Hacking 1990; Packard 1989, 1997a; Scott 1999).

In contrast, postwar postcolonial health development efforts were born in part as a critique of these regimes, and, to some extent, they reformulated the possibilities of intervention in and around the birth of the postcolonial nation-state as a *response* to empire (Bose 1997; Nandy 1989; Stepan 2011). Multilateral and bilateral forms of health aid that came into being after World War II continued to count things like the spread of disease, the loss of productivity to disease, population health, and public health, but, in the aftermath of empires, they increasingly had to do so in relation to the unit of the nation state (through national ministries of health that were tasked with producing national health statistics; Greene 2008; Rees 2014).

In fact, organizations like the World Health Organization (WHO) often struggled to forge a path that transcended national interests (Chorev 2012), even while newly independent nations strove to assert claims to independence in part through health and health care (Osseo-Asare 2014). So while postwar institutions that grew in the decades after decolonization believed in a transcendent form of policymaking in which *international* bodies would set aside their national interests and create a world in which a flourishing economy could produce an even playing field, where distributions of the world's health (and health care resources) would be equitable across nations, and where the possibilities for another world war would be reduced (Finnemore 1997; Staples 2006), this process was often fraught with political divides between North and South, poor and wealthy, socialist and capitalist nations (Chorev 2012). Their worldwide goals, in part, resurrected those of earlier pan-state health agencies (such as those at the International Sanitary Convention in Paris in 1851 or at agencies like the Pan American Health Organization, founded in 1902) in their desires for international health equity in relation to both controlling the spread of disease and/or eradication of them (Stepan 2011). Even when these postwar institutions were organized around the principle of "one nation, one vote" (as the WHO was), Chorev (2012) reminds us that national concerns remained more visible than ever and, in fact, had to be managed carefully. Global health, as we will see, attempts, or imagines, something new.

Continuity and rupture over this early transition from colonial to postcolonial public health can also be traced in relation to how these eras and institutions envisioned the relationships between health and economics. Colonial health programs gave birth to statistics practices that configured population health in relation to colonial economies. Even colonial-era missionaries and humanitarian organizations were, in their own ways, focused in some measure on counting things, even if it was "souls saved" as much as "laboring bodies" (Brown 1979; Packard 1989; Rose Hunt 1999; Stepan

2011; Vaughan 2001). Health was also intertwined with practices that exceeded economics, such as when it enabled the colonized, or the postcolonial, to serve as a subject of science (Anderson 2006; Prakash 1999; Tilley 2011) and when it was authorized by and configured as humanitarian service (Birn 2014; Brown 1976, 1979; Chandler 2001). Counting health here often meant calibrating the impact to extractive industries due to things like tuberculosis, malaria, hookworm, even infertility (Brown 1979; Packard 1989, 2011; Rose Hunt 1999).

In the postwar postcolonial era efforts to control or eradicate disease and distribute health resources shifted the priorities between health and economics. If the health of natives was important to colonial administrators because of the need for labor in colonial industries even when carried out under the guise of benevolence, then in the postcolonial postwar era the assumption early on was that the health aspired to through development programs was of value in its own right (and that, indeed, impoverishment from colonial labor was often to blame for poor health). Still, in postwar international health work it was often assumed that health could be achieved only *through* simultaneous economic development, that with economic development health improvements would follow seamlessly (Bose 1997; Farley 2003; Packard 1997a, 1997b). In the cold war environment, the focus on economic development over other routes to health sometimes masked and at other times exacerbated larger debates over the benefits of socialism versus capitalism in provisioning "health for all."

The blurred lines of cause and effect between health and economic development (that is, over whether to conceptualize health or economics as the top priority) at places like the Rockefeller Foundation (long before the postwar era) were inherited by many international health institutions that aimed to accomplish what colonial medicine failed to accomplish — namely to eradicate diseases and bring health to the natives (Birn 2014; Farley 2006; Stepan 2011). But even where the cause-and-effect relations between economic and health goals were reversed, the grand arc of health development (from colonial times through the postwar era) demonstrates a striking persistence of thinking in more foundational ways about health in terms of human productivity in economic terms.

One might argue that in the postwar era the shifting links between health and economic development priorities became more troublesome than ever, forming a source of extraordinary tension and debate within multilateral institutions like the WHO and in the various bilateral aid agencies. One could even talk about shifts in postwar international health policy solely in relation to these battles between economics and health. The political economic assumptions of the Alma Ata Summit and the primary health care movement are often set against the policies of structural adjustment programs as both political economic agendas forged paths through the half-century of cold war diplomacy (Chorev 2012). Still, at the end of the day, these debates have frequently dissolved into just that: combat over one kind of political-economic policy versus another in relation to health policy. Seldom have international health institutions been able to sustain the more bold (some would say naïve) mission of promising health as a human right, regardless of cost or any particular political-economic theory.

In sum, how postwar world health institutions have gone about measuring things in relation to health is in some part continuous with efforts seen during the colonial era and in some part quite different. Efforts to eradicate diseases in the colonial epoch were largely replicated in early postwar institutions (Farley 2003; Packard 1997a, 1997b, 2011; Stepan 2011) and reproduced many of the debates over the links between economics and health. At the same time, concerns over health under empire were supplanted in the postcolonial era by concerns over health conceptualized in and through the nation-state. Similarly some of the links between economics and health configured under colonialism became reconstituted in the postwar period in policies that linked health development to economic development, even while new formulations of "health as a right" were augmented. All of these efforts and transitions were accompanied by ways of counting that fit the administrative and worldly aspirations of these times.

In contrast, *global health* is often construed as having the capacity (and focus) to transcend both the nation-state and the endless deliberation over which politics best serve to advance health in relation to economic development. Not surprisingly, it also imagines having the ability to count things differently. This is explored more fully in chapter 1. Briefly, however, the shift away from national-level discourse is in part because of the crisis resulting from the decline of fiscal support from national entities (Birn 2014; McGoey et al. 2011) and from the growing sentiment that national entities often *get in the way* of effective health delivery rather than promoting it. This latter sentiment is nested inside more critical perspectives from within global health institutions today that conceptualize both disease and interventions in ways that are believed to transcend national boundaries because they are not "political" (Rees 2014). This has not, however, entailed transcending thinking of health in and through economics or economical ways of counting, as we will see.

Global health is thus imagined as a rubric for doing something that has not been done before: to imagine health in a truly global way, to do health work in ways that are not dependent upon the nation-state and, as we will see, that put the old stale debates over economics and politics to rest. Global health planners envision a world of diseases constantly in motion, always on the move to new places without regard to nation-state capacities and limitations. Global health professionals also envision a world in which interventions can be mapped out as problems of scale and measurement (or specifically as counting practices) rather than as problems of custom, culture, or national political will. The dominant discourses in global health today also imagine a world in which neoliberal economic strategies will seamlessly work toward the achievement of health as a right of, and therefore achievable for, all. What enables all this to happen today, of course, is metrics.

Today key institutions of global health such as the Global Fund, the Bill and Melinda Gates Foundation, and the Institute on Health Metrics and Evaluation all envision using a form of global knowledge that is based on universals (biology, disease, vaccines, etc.), in which multiplicity is visible only in and through global (that is, universal) forms of data production that get lumped together as "metrics." Metrics are technologies of counting, but specifically technologies of counting that form global knowledge. Metrics used today are imagined to offer uniform and standardized conversations about how best to intervene, how best to conceptualize health and disease, how best to both count and be accountable, and how best to pay for it all.

One of the goals of this volume is to explore how global health metrics pose a problem of knowledge in relation to our understanding of not only the past but also the future or what might be called *global health efficacy*. Specifically, how do counting efforts seen in the turn to randomized controlled trials (RCTs), and its related forms of evidence-based practice, become the new arbiters of what counts in relation to health outcomes? How does the demand for counting in these ways impact what health workers do? How do efforts to produce RCT-like statistical validity get undermined by more basic problems of counting births, deaths, disease, and morbidity at all? How do these challenges pose problems for nation-states, for local, regional, or national governments?

The chapters here provide evidence that global health metrics enable and encourage efforts to produce health in ways that sometimes work well and sometimes do not. We witness celebration of *the new* coupled with frequent exasperation over the recurring sense that *we have been here before.* Indeed global knowledge is fraught with many of the same problems of inclusion and exclusion (of evidence, people, problems) that were seen in the era of colonialism and in the era of postwar development aid. Still the metrics of global health authorize new demands for all of us involved in this work, and they produce effects far beyond their specific numbers. These demands and effects can be read in relation to debates about sovereignty.

Metrics and Sovereignty

What do health workers do when they cannot produce the kinds of numbers that give statistically robust results? What do they do when deaths mess up the numbers needed to claim health program success? What light do these activities and failures shed on the ways sovereignty and global health metrics work together today? The push for better ways of counting and better indices of accountability in what has been called evidence-based medicine is not new (as chapter 1 will discuss). However, the call for such tactics in global health today seems to often rely on a kind of forgetfulness, or perhaps a studied ignorance, of the past and the many efforts to critique these tactics in the Global North.

To the extent that expectations for metrics are promoted today at the largest institutions for health aid, and to the extent that funding for global health work is increasingly tied to these metrics, we explore in this volume the way the effort to "do metrics" contributes to forms of sovereignty that may ultimately challenge older forms of political sovereignty that emerged in the postwar era. Thus if we think of sovereignty in relation to the mid-seventeenth-century notion of Westphalian territorial governance, then what do we call it when a sovereign nation's ability to govern becomes increasingly dominated not just by the regimes of development aid that reiterated its national borders (indeed its right to national forms of knowledge) but by those that aim to transcend these borders? This volume begins to answer this question or, at least, opens that conversation.

In his 1999 book, *Seeing Like the State*, James Scott noted that the degree to which modern governments succeed or fail depends in part on their ability to create systems of quantification that render complex social phenomena comparable and countable. Postcolonial international health could be seen as having given rise to quantification practices that leveraged the use of international resources for state building. Metrics-driven political economic arrangements today, however, may promote infringements on state sovereignty in and through global health regimes. The degree to which these forms of counting ironically reproduce older forms seen under colonialism is a concern here. The wide range of phenomena that are pushed inside and outside of visibility in the wake of the demand for metrics, and how these acts of recognition, exclusion, and inclusion draw our attention to problems of not only epistemology and economics but also politics and governance are all important. This volume provides studies in the trials and tribulations of a multidisciplinary effort to *do global health through metrics* but also opens the conversation about what else is at stake in these efforts in relation to an aspirational postcolonial, but also post international health — that is, post–nation-state — form of global health sovereignty.

The use of the term *metrics* in this volume is itself somewhat aspirational. Our papers suggest that the ideal form of metrics used in accounting today in global health programs is in fact often more hoped-for than achieved. Indeed the counting practices of today are as troubled by imperfection as were the efforts in previous times. This does not, however, get in the way of efforts to produce them, nor does it impede efforts to rely on their empirical products as if they were indelibly factual. One of the attractions of metrics is their ability to hold status as apolitical or politically neutral forms of evidence. Of course, no history of metrics would suggest that counting exercises are not deeply entangled with politics. Still, the assumption still seems to be in many global health circles that numbers will offer unbiased, apolitical truths about health outcomes or health conditions. Our focus here, on the specific kinds of metrics that are espoused at today's global health institutions and in global health efforts all over the world, is to trace these productivities and to specify how they conceal, reveal, and generate both success and failure when it comes to problems of both politics and health.

The authors here note that not only are reliable numbers both frequently impossible to get and frequently misleading in the world of global health but also that other forms of evidence may be *more* reliable than those that can be rendered through metrics. Getting the empirical facts needed for metrics may entail a kind of violence to the empirical truths they aim to produce. Other kinds of evidence may be more reliable than numbers. In this sense, quantification strategies and the metrics we rely on to *avoid* politics often do not avoid politics at all; they become a form of politics in their own right, augmenting the political stakes and political underpinnings of health projects in a manner that is frequently invisible to those who believe in these exercises in calculation and counting. In this sense the notion that metrics are not (and never have been) politically neutral is not only worth repeating, but also exploring further.

Most of us (and certainly not only anthropologists) know that numbers are never intrinsically capable of proving anything; they must be made to speak in very specific ways about what they claim to represent (Crump 1990). In fact we might see number crunching and metrics work as, in their own way, forms of storytelling. They tell stories about what those who produce them and what those who rely on them care about most. These cares are coded into the naming of some variables as important and the exclusion of others, as Bowker and Star (1999) have shown. They are coded into the statistical forms of reason that are thought to produce facts about which interventions worked and which interventions failed, the causes of death, cost effectiveness, and on and on. This is more than saying metrics are politically coded or that numbers can decide fates (of individuals or whole populations) as, at one time, only sovereigns could. Specific numbers can certainly move policy, confer political allegiance, guarantee funding, even bring about health. But they do so not simply by claiming truth about the empirical world. They do so because of the ways they are "produced" and the ways they are circulated. These productivities and circulations are the stories that precede and exceed numerical forms of truth-telling. At the same time, metrical forms of reason, and truth-telling often displace other kinds of knowledge, other forms of evidence (Sangaramoorthy and Benton 2012). Metzl (2010) reminds us that metrical forms of reason and accountability can both conceal and produce empirical facts that work against health. We further this project by studying how producing metrical forms of accountability can displace other activities, other ways of knowing, and other ways of seeing, seeing other things. These are the other kinds of stories that metrics tell.

Similarly, while it is commonplace to fall back on the truism that numbers are inherently *not neutral* in that they can always *be used* for any political purpose, as many authors have shown, it is another thing to show how the act of data collection becomes always and invariably political as a form of knowledge *because* it claims political neutrality. In fact, it takes a lot of work to make something seem politically "neutral," especially when this assumption undergirds efforts to actually *make* political claims or to set political cal policy. When the WHO uses metrics to push back on health-jeopardizing political policies (advancing a pro-health politics of their own), they do so by presuming the truthfulness of numbers in and of themselves (Chorev 2012), and this takes a lot of work and a lot of management of evidence in such a way that the numbers do this political work. How metrics, as forms of evidence-making, constitute a politics in their own right by claiming neutrality still needs to be explored ethnographically. Anthropologists, long concerned with the problems of veridication in and around different kinds of evidence (Leibow et al. 2013), have returned to this exploration today by looking at quantification and its epistemic demands on reason and on practice. Our book extends this project by exploring how the production of metrics works in global health today as a political imperative tied to new forms of evidence, old statistical forms of reason, painfully lingering financial arrangements of neoliberalism, and disruptions of notions of national sovereignty that have become visible in our time.

I do not mean by this that numbers can never be helpful to the project of health. On the contrary, the assumption is usually that numbers and the metrics they sustain are needed for improved health and health care policy. But, as scholars like Jean Lave (1988) and Helen Verran (2001) have shown, even the basic notion of counting (long before it is rendered "scientific") needs to be seen as a learned, culturally specific possibility. People not only count in different ways; they also take counting to mean different things. Why, then, would we assume that the turn to using statistical forms of reasoning since the nineteenth century in order to make sense of social life has been anything but similarly conditional on certain very specific, colonial, postcolonial, and sometimes very neocolonial kinds of arrangements, as Hacking (1990) notes? Similarly we might interrogate how the metrics being pushed today (in relation to statistics, RCTs, and evidence-based medicine) are also conditional on specific political and economic arrangements that hope to transcend old politics and political forms.

As the use of quantitative forms of reasoning has grown in the health and clinical sciences since the nineteenth century, so too has it become harder and harder to imagine that these forms of managing the empirical world are simply artifacts of culture or politics. But they are. Their spread and their refinement during the second half of the so-called postcolonial century and their growth and acceptance as useful to the work of global health in the first decades of the new millennium have gone unchallenged in too many global health circles. They are not entirely unchallenged, and many of those who work in and through these forms of reason (including economists and statisticians) have debated the utility of one kind of accounting over another, as we will see. Still the rolling out of expectations around statistical and experimental forms of data and evidence has been consistently growing in ways that deserve more scrutiny.

Ethnography

Anthropologists have been saying a lot about these trends in general, and medical anthropology has much to add to this conversation in global health in particular. The chapters here document the specific ways practices of *inventory* and *intervention* through metrics work in detail in global health. As RCTs and statistically robust forms of health work become the gold standard for not only showing effectiveness but also for obtaining funding, so too do these techniques become pathways for other things: for getting elected to political office, for asserting native sovereignty, for making profits.

At the same time, these chapters suggest that the metrics, even while being produced, often produce collateral effects and opportunities that mess up our easy confidence in the numbers. In fact they show that ethnographic research — because it enables a focus on single cases in all of their singular and idiosyncratic complexity but also because it enables a focus on other kinds of evidence writ large — produces empirical data that form not only an evidence base but an evidence base that is sometimes more truthful, proposing alternatives to the evidence-making from metrics work. Ethnographic materials are a potential source of alternative evidence that not only contrasts with the kinds of evidence required for good metrics work but also sometimes unseats its hold on truth.

The metrics of concern in these chapters appear in many ethnographic forms. Sometimes they refer to numerical accountabilities over how many women died or lived after giving birth, and sometimes they refer to more complex modes of numerical figuring: RCTs, power calculations, other kinds of statistics, other kinds of counting. Always the need for numerical data appears as a kind of burden of proof, as if proof lay intrinsically in what the numbers tell us. Each chapter offers evidence about how metrical forms of reason get tangled up in things far beyond health, while preventing other specificities of health to be concealed. Cumulatively we might say that these stories tell us something about how the new commitments to metrics both work and don't work in the effort to do global health today.

Finally, what can be made of the stories — the empirical events, experiences, and myriad occurrences and facts — that do not lend themselves to being counted, or at least not counted without an epistemological violence being done to the complicated empirical truths they offer? What are we to do with empirical truths about particularities and interwoven strands of cause and effect, of rationality, that seem always beyond the pale of reductive forms of counting — the things that spill over and can't be included in the counting exercises?

For some it is the hallmark of the ethnographic method to try to capture the vast breadth and depth of this complexity of the singular case. The goal is often to capture this complexity without reducing the phenomena observed to simple forms that can be counted in ways that make one case just like another, one specific event comparable to the next. Forms of knowledge that resist reductionism, for many an anthropologist, provide more stable and more reliable forms of truth-telling than those that involve reductionism. But what of the fact that many of us (I would guess), if faced with the opportunity to ensure a single life was saved or to document that a single intervention worked, would still want to "count" this as important enough to change policy, to change the world, even if it carried no statistical or metrical weight of validity? How can we count these complex and singular experiential moments in ways that do not involve reductions in the march toward better metrics in global health? Might these sorts of facts work as a form of affective accountability for metrics exercises, or might they instead work to unseat the claims of the metrics, or might they do both?

The Chapters

Metrics trends in international health have a long history, but it has been only in recent decades, and with the arrival of what is being called *global health*, that a new kind of metrics has been promoted as the sine qua non — an indispensable ingredient — of good global health work. In part I, "Getting Good Numbers," Claire Wendland and Adeola Oni-Orisan show how the effort to produce numbers for global health statistics is deeply fraught. Both are looking at the case of maternal mortality in African states; both make it very clear that the counting practices used to make claims about successes and failures in maternal health often place political outcomes over those of health.

Wendland reveals with stunning clarity how statistical accounts of maternal mortality in Malawi enable the production of truths that not only distort empirical reality through estimation practices but also efface massive amounts of information about who is involved with and what really happens during deliveries on the ground. Taking us on an ethnographic tour from the clinic to the world forums where maternal mortality statistics are used to justify state budgets and election campaigns, but also through the statistical forgeries that provide a lexicon for such activities, Wendland reveals the logics that enable conversations about death rates to feel real and solid even while necessarily being deeply flawed. She shows us how important these numbers are and how they become authorized as arbiters of action, even while documenting how hard it is to get "real" numbers that nevertheless must be produced because they serve so many different purposes.

Oni-Orisan reveals similar problems in the production of statistics about maternal mortality in Nigeria. Starting in the clinic and observing a case of maternal death "erasure," she asks: How does the production of numbers depend on the political accomplishments that those numbers promise? Tracing the effects of the metrics from the invisibilities they leave behind, Oni-Orisan is able to show that numbers are not simply tools used in the political rhetoric of aspiring state bureaucrats; they are enactments of politics in their own right. Political careers are made and destroyed by way of health statistics in this region of Nigeria. Recognized as a global health success by funding agencies that are deeply invested in metrics, health aid becomes a new kind of tool for governance, and political legitimacy trickles down to decision-making and accounting practices at the hospital bedside. These practices, she notes, can mean political success, even when they result in unnecessary mortalities that remain hidden.

Over time and with enough evidence like this, we start to see a picture of omission and erasure—lives that are not saved, programs that have been derailed—that accompany or are enabled by the reliance on metrics. This is a problem not just in one place, with one aberrant program here and there. This is a problem found in many places, in many instances, where numbers are demanded. Exploring the production of numbers up close like this enables one to begin to see their solidity dissolve. Stories about this produce a form of counterevidence and this is a good place to begin this volume.

Part II, "Metrics Politics," tackles thorny questions about how metrics become integral to practices of governance in the postcolonial era. That is, whereas part I affirmed the ways numbers and their production are political acts, part II explores how metrics become tangled up in state governance and problems of sovereignty. Marlee Tichenor offers a stunning example of this in her study of the data-retention strike in Senegal, in which health workers made citizenship demands on the state (for better pay, working conditions, etc.) by withholding data that the state needed to make its claims about health and budgets for aid. Although we are shown in this chapter not only how "wobbly" the numbers are (as Wendland calls them) because of the conditions of their production, Tichenor also shows us how solid they must be made to seem because of their foundational role in governance in states like Senegal, where large sectors of the economy are tied to the health sector.

In a similar vein Molly Hales shows us how metrics activity becomes entangled in problematic ways with efforts to assert sovereignty on the part of Native Alaskan Yup'ik. She points to the messiness that arises from efforts to document efficacy using metrics, particularly in the case of Native American sovereignty that for at least a few decades has pushed for use of tribal concepts of ethics, health, and community as a basis for designing health interventions and treatments. As Native Alaskan Yup'ik sovereignty shifted in the 1970s toward architectures of neoliberalism, the question of how tribal sovereignty is enacted in this region is doubly vexed by being beholden to fiscal priorities (the tribe must be run at least in part like a business) but also to the problems of funding public sector activities that cannot pay for themselves. In Hales's pithy explication of these dynamics, we learn of tensions that bubble up over how to manage the production of evidence when the stakes of using some kinds of evidence over others are deeply tied to the very vision of sovereignty (and the fiscal tactics used for this) that locals care the most about.

In part III, "Metrics Economics," Susan Erikson and Lily Walkover offer compelling evidence that the burdens of a new emphasis on metrics are meted out in and through complex orchestrations of finance, producing accountabilities that are as much about fiscal profit and survival as they are about health. Erikson begins with a scathing exploration of the linkages between creative financing and profit-driven solutions that are being pushed by the big players in global health funding today, teasing out the threads that have sutured together corporate interests and investment models to the humanitarian work of global health. Walking in step with my own exploration in chapter one, Erikson takes us down into the nitty-gritty details of these neoliberal relationships. New partnerships between public and private entities, investment portfolios and humanitarian missions, profit-making and health outcomes are all enabled by the use of metrics, and the particular fiscal architectures that are being celebrated up the line by global health planners and financiers become highly questionable in a number of ways. When funds for health programs are derived by way of investments in companies that are also responsible for disease, we might question whether this arrangement is truly a win-win arrangement. Perhaps unraveling the role of metrics in all this will help us to unravel, or at least make visible, what is at stake in some of the more questionable practices in this set of arrangements.

In affirmation of the cartography of market-driven global health mapped out by Erikson, Walkover offers a troubling example of the outcomes of metrics-driven demands at a nonprofit. She also suggests an opportunity to think of how to change the discourse. Hesperian Health Guides, which has arguably made one of the largest impacts in global health over the entire era of postcolonial health development through its *Where There Is No Doctor* books, confronts the new demands for metrics, the same metrics Erikson points to in her study of finance in global health. Walkover shows how these demands put organizations like Hesperian at risk. By tracing the organizations' ethos and practices that have traditionally been grassroots and bottom-up in ways that do not easily lend themselves to being statistically countable, Walkover maps out exactly what is at stake in trying to meet the demand for new metrics data. In searching for better metrics as evidence of their success, the very practices that have made these organizations successful are often derailed. Remaining accountable to communities is often undermined by requests to make communities "countable" for the benefit of potential funders.

Part IV, "Storied Metrics," thus explores the proposition that is implicit in the chapters up to this point: that we might read the metrics as storied in their own ways. However, the chapters here tell us a good deal about how people working within metrics systems work against the idea that metrics tell only one kind of story. Carolyn Smith-Morris takes up the issue of "fidelity" that is used in metrics work as a form of veridication (establishing that the data are reliable because they were collected with fidelity to the protocol). Looking at how ethnographers worked with RCT research on veterans with spinal cord injuries in the U.S. Veterans Hospital Administration, Smith-Morris shows that achieving fidelity does not necessarily mean that RCT work is capturing the kind of evidence that actually reveals why the program works or does not work. Efforts often fail to capture these messy and uncountable details that really make a difference in veterans' lives. Still, she shows, statistical accounts are used to move policy forward and to justify one kind of program over others. Her work suggests that statistical practices might actually be read as social processes and entanglements that enable these programs to claim success and also constitute their existential power on the ground, in the clinic. How researchers like Smith-Morris, who are on the front lines of RCT anthropological engagements in health care, are actually interrogating and changing the work of RCT metrics is a topic we have much to learn from in relation to critique and also in relation to productive opportunities. This work, she implies, forms a different lexicon for speaking not only about outcomes but also about fidelity in research.

Another way to think about the storied metrics of global health is through what Pierre Minn offers; he shows that as global health interventions are increasingly expressed in terms of quantitative outcomes and "deliverables," individuals and organizations whose activities fall outside the purview of these units must find ways to communicate their actions to funders and supporters, a theme also touched on in Hales's and Walkover's chapters. Studying Konbit Sante, a U.S.-based NGO working in northern Haiti whose mandate explicitly eschews clinical interventions and the development of a "parallel health system," Minn illustrates how staff and volunteers draw on the language of alterity and distinction to gain visibility and support for their programs. The organization's emphasis on the relational aspects of their work has proven to be a double-edged sword, both limiting opportunities for expansion while earning them a prominent reputation among actors in Haiti's health sector. As they work to represent their accomplishments in the quantified terms that meet the demands of transnational aid bureaucracies ("widgets") in ways that resonate with the affective sensibilities of individual North American donors, they also accomplish a kind of global health that speaks back to power in and through a critical engagement with metrics.

As closure for the volume, I offer a brief epilogue that takes up the question of what counts as good global health work under the pressures of global health metrics today. Instead of reiterating the flaws of metrical forms of accountability, I discuss a few novel propositions being put forth by colleagues and practitioners who are in their own ways toying with the problem of numbers and answering those who question the tendency toward tyranny in the global health conversations we are having. Overall my hope is that readers will be called to consider how else we might think about the architectures of global health in terms of who benefits and who does not, about what we mean by evidence in the steady march toward better forms of accountability, and to embrace the possibility of plural forms of deliberation over what we mean by both evidence and efficacy at all in global health.

1 · METRICS OF THE GLOBAL SOVEREIGN

Numbers and Stories in Global Health VINCANNE ADAMS

Universalism

The second half of the nineteenth century was a heady time, especially for those who believed that if you had the right metrics, you could rule the world. Nowhere was this more visible than when (as the *Economist* notes) "those two great imperial rivals, Britain and France, agreed to carve up not merely the world, but the Universe." In 1847 "the British gained control of time, which is why the Earth's prime meridian . . . runs through Greenwich, a suburb of London. [Thirty years later], the French annexed length and mass. They kept them, in the form of two lumps of metal, in sealed jars in [the Bureau of Weights and Measures] in Sevres, a suburb of Paris."[1]

The idea of creating universal standards of measurement was arguably more than a practical solution to the needs of maritime trade and currency exchange that calibrated the colonial enterprises of those times. Universal standards required fundamentally new ways of thinking about objectivity itself (as Daston and Galison 2010 have noted). Objectivity, in its own way, served as the invented conceptual counterpart to the hubris of the age of imperialism. It was joined over roughly the same decades by the birth of statistics, the overachieving mathematical offspring of universally standardized time, mass, and weight.[2]

The creation of these systems of counting in relation to standardized notions of measurement enabled a practical set of tools for colonial rule, working to ensure the smooth transition from mercantilism to direct and indirect systems of colonial governance. Historians of science also note that the metrics were a morally aspirational undertaking: they offered the possibility of shared conversations and shared bases for comparison, for evaluation, for stabilizing the truth around complex assemblages of people, life, and nature, and for creating policies for governing that took ethical questions out of the hands of the priests and colonial rulers and put them into the morally neutral hands of scientifically minded experts.[3] Universal metrics offered, in short, new ways of stabilizing the randomness and chaos produced by the violence of colonialism (Scott 1999).

For this reason it is sometimes hard to remember that despite the aspirational opportunities they afforded, *universal standards* presupposed a unity of purpose and desire for such standards rather than the recognition that, in fact, in order to be "universal" these standards had to be forced upon the world. Their universality, like their objectivity, had to be taught and learned and forged in a crucible of colonial occupations, sometimes against the backdrop of a good deal of resistance and against the hardship of ever new demands on subjective experience (Anderson 2006; Harding 1998; Packard 1989; Rose Hunt 1999; Scott 1999; Vaughan 2001).

Ruptures and Continuities: From Colonial to Postwar International Health Aid to Global Health

The persistence of universal standards into the twentieth century reveals an equal persistence of aspirations that had to be sustained and relearned in the postwar postcolonial era as formerly colonized nations found themselves both liberated and subjugated in new ways. Resurrected over the century that witnessed colonialism's decline, universal standards of measurement and audit were redeployed and reinvented by economists and politicians and formed into architectures of debt and finance that transformed former colonies into recipients of development aid.

Laboring under the universal obligation to adopt a "will to improve"

(Murray Li 2007), as "modern believers" (Pigg 1996), or, now, as "trauma portfolio" managers (James 2010), the world's postcolonial poor have over and over again been taught to imagine themselves as needy subjects, as targets of intervention, as hygienic, nutrition-conscious, clinic-seeking, safe-motherhood-striving, and, now, data-producing, entrepreneurial global citizens (Escobar 1994, Ferguson 2006). Never mind that just committing to these identities was not enough then and remains never enough (even when inhabited) for the vast majority of the poorest of the poor to achieve health and well-being; today whole nations have been, by design, kept alive — or at least barely alive and (in the eyes of the cynics) always needing more — in and through these conduits of financial and development aid. Third world debt economies have always relied on the ongoing displacements entailed in the fact that aid seldom eliminates problems of neediness, and the endless effort to configure newer and better ways of intervening to fix the problems of neediness remains ongoing. As a result governments have sometimes been entirely remade to accommodate the protean agendas of donor nations in order to obtain aid, and, in turn, they have participated in new regimes of sovereignty, which, I would argue, still have everything to do with measuring things.

International health development, for its part, has formed one pillar of the postcolonial mosaic at the ever more sensitive sites of bodies, sickness, and death. But if colonial efforts to count things in health imagined no borders, the aftermath of empire witnessed the opposite in the burgeoning form of the nation-state. Even when the *worldly* aspirations of international health policies were achieved at places like the World Health Organization (who), knowing how to implement these policies and how to *count* their successes and failures was now something that had to be done through national ministries of health, national statistics, and national politics (Chorev 2012; Greene 2008; Rees 2014).

OTHER THINGS REMAINED constant across the colonial-postcolonial divide, including the tangled interdependencies of health and economics. Thus it is clear that while international public health agencies early on offered an antidote to colonialism's rapacious capitalism, they also helped to secure its operations over time.[4] Being globally poor and needy, or healthy, in the six-decade-long era of health development has always entailed and still entails being a conduit for servicing debt and the circulations of capital that this debt allows. These figurations of debt and subjectivity are deeply tied to the use of metrics.

Like the Hindu deity Vishnu, postcolonial health aid might be seen as a being with many arms doing different kinds of things frequently marked by the dual (and competing, even anachronistic) logics of the Washington consensus and its critics—racketing between Friedman's neoliberal policies and Keynesian welfare policies as they are interpreted by health aid organizations. This Vishnu offers two arms to treat malaria and two to sell pesticides; two arms to make motherhood safe and two to sell contraception; two arms to build low-cost latrines and two to convince people to use costly hospitals; two to mix up the oral rehydration solution and another two to sell the essential drugs that would displace these simple remedies.[5]

Not infrequently, it has been the careening back and forth between competing policies that is blamed for the lack of significant progress in international health. The truth is, it is hard to tell which politics (and economics) are actually to blame: Is structural adjustment to blame for having derailed the public health agendas of the 1970s? Or is it structural adjustment's reason for being—ongoing poverty, the poverty that has remained despite twenty years of international health efforts—that was and is to blame, demanding, more aid, more loans and now market solutions (Ferguson 2006)? That is, the displacement of the leftist and liberal-leaning Alma Ata (and the primary health care movement) policies by more conservative policies (the World Bank's growing interest in health, its production of the World Development Report in 1993, structural adjustment and, later, the UN Millennium Development Goals, MDGs) only partly defines the problem we face today, only partially explains the failures.[6]

I would argue that postwar policymakers and their critics have often had in common the fact that no matter which side of the political divide they are on (Keynes vs. Friedman, Sachs vs. Easterly), they seem to agree that economics remains the centerpiece and central solution for all things health backward. One finds, in other words, a persistent reduction of health inequality to problems of economic lack, a focus that returns once again, like the circling vulture above its already dead prey, to problems of politics. Often this politics underpins another, in which the blame for lack of health development progress is shifted onto the nation-state itself, in rhetorics of political will and corruption, which, again, returns us to questions of competing politics over carrots versus sticks in development aid.[7]

Not surprisingly global health arrives as a clarion call for something new and transcendent. Global health calls for something that will transcend politics altogether. What it calls for is better metrics. Metrics, it seems, are the panacea we've all been waiting for. Metrics will, once and for all, get us talking about evidence instead of politics. Metrics today are assumed to be able to give us a value-neutral, but also politically unbiased, way of talking about health problems and their solutions.[8] Nowhere is this more visible than in the latest iteration of grand international health policy called "Global Health 2035: A World Converging within a Generation" (also called the "Grand Convergence" for short; Jamison et al. 2015) where entire health systems are conceptualized as problems that can be solved using the metrics tools of health economics. Thus the trend over time has not been simply away from liberal toward conservative thinking but rather more simply toward the market overall or, as I will show, toward letting the economists do our thinking for us. And how do economists think? Through numbers.

Indeed it seems that today doing global health means caring an awful lot about the numbers.[9] Being able to count what it is we are doing seems to matter more than ever before, and so we participate in ever more sophisticated forms of audit, research, and accounting that are rolled out, chi-squared, and scaled up. The Millennium Development Goals might be hard to reach, but it is not hard to see that the only way to know if we have reached them is if we have good ways of measuring the outcomes of what we are doing now.[10] At stake here, as it was in the nineteenth century, is how to find a metric that can serve as a universal standard.

Measuring Life, Getting to Global Health

In the annual letter from the Bill and Melinda Gates Foundation (2013), Bill Gates opens his report by noting one of the most important problems facing global health programs today:

> Over the holidays, I read *The Most Powerful Idea in the World*, a brilliant chronicle by William Rosen of the many innovations it took to harness steam power. Among the most important were a new way to measure the energy output of engines and a micrometer dubbed the "Lord Chancellor," able to gauge tiny distances.
>
> Such measuring tools . . . allowed inventors to see if their incre-

mental design changes led to the improvements — higher-quality parts, better performance, and less coal consumption — needed to build better engines. Innovations in steam power demonstrate a larger lesson: Without feedback from precise measurement . . . invention is "doomed to be rare and erratic." With it, invention becomes "commonplace."

Of course, the work of our foundation is a world away from the making of steam engines. But in the past year I have been struck again and again by how important measurement is to improving the human condition. You can achieve amazing progress if you set a clear goal and find a measure that will drive progress toward that goal — in a feedback loop similar to the one Rosen describes. This may seem pretty basic, but it is amazing to me how often it is not done and how hard it is to get right.

If Gates is even close to being right that doing better global health is at least kind of like building a steam engine, then this proposition is, as he says, based on the challenge of building the right kind of instrument for measuring things. His aspiration is both noble and practical, built on the dual desires to rectify problems of health inequality and to use science and technology to do so. But how does one kind of measuring system get chosen over others? That the micrometer was dubbed the "Lord Chancellor" is not to be missed. Just as the Lord Chancellor enabled the steam engine to bring us into the industrial era, we now hope for a new kind of Lord Chancellor that will bring us into a postdevelopment world in which some form of "health for all" will finally be achieved.[11]

Gates is not alone in hoping for a new Lord Chancellor, or what might be called *one metric to rule them all*. An entire community of emergent global health scholars declares that the commitment to health for all is possible only through ever more complex transformations in the practices of producing and navigating the metrics. Most of the leading textbooks on global health, for instance, focus in their first chapters on measurements and metrics.

A recent installment of the *Lancet*'s coverage of global health, devoted specifically to a conference on global health metrics sponsored by the University of Washington, offers a version of this too.[12] By using better metrics, global health advocates hope that we will set stale political debates to rest and will also get our focus back on what really matters: health.[13] More important, perhaps, we will stop wasting money on interventions that apparently don't work and put more money into those that do, or at least those that promise to work better.

The proliferation of conversations about metrics is tied to other transformations and experiments in how to do health work in the global context and how to pay for it. The "postwar pocket," to borrow a phrase from Jean-Paul Gaudilliere, that grew public multilateral and bilateral institutions committed to state funding for international health development has been shrinking. Indeed if colonial-era health development relied on a mixture of humanitarian, foundation, and missionary efforts working in tandem with colonial and imperialistic government agendas (Brown 1976, 1979; Packard 1997b; Palmer 2010), then the postcolonial development era and its birth of large multilateral institutions for health governance and assistance corralled public resources in unprecedented ways, to some extent limiting the power of the private sector or tethering it to the consensual models of the multilateral *public* institution.

Today, however, we witness a return to private sector NGO and humanitarian organizations as the institutional forms of choice for doing global health work.[14] Global health today has become a platform that binds the public and private sector interests in novel form, inheriting the common sense of neoliberalism and increasingly mobilizing the private sector and its market-based, profit-driven solutions for all health problems. Old debates over carrots versus sticks have been all but abandoned today for models of aid and development that mix charity and profit, making carrots and sticks part of the same agenda. The public-private alliances emerging in global health that use these tactics, I argue, are now being conceptualized in and through new ways of counting and new languages of metrics. Metrics not only enable us to set aside questions of politics; they also turn moral questions (about these blurrings) into problems of numbers. It is thus no surprise that the Gates Foundation is the one funding both the Institute for Health Metrics and Evaluation (with the University of Washington) and the Health Metrics Network in Geneva (Erikson, this volume). The rise in involvement of private sector corporations and foundations and the subtle ways they tie market interests to health outcomes may make us pause to consider how these might return us to the specter of empire. Still the route to this end point is not direct.

The story of economics metrics in postwar international health is complicated. There were early discussions that borrowed heavily not only from colonial health efforts but also from public health in the developed world. These included lengthy debates over how to count complex phenomena in relation to cost of investment in health, including how to measure the behavior of publics, the conditions of labor, and the spread of disease, particularly in England. Efforts by scholars such as Archie Cochrane, and Ian and Tom Chalmers led to the birth of clinical epidemiology and the perception that one could use robust statistical methods of randomization and evaluation to determine effectiveness of interventions (Daly 2005). Conversations like this continued in the early postwar era of international health as they were brought to bear on efforts to eradicate infectious and tropical diseases through multilateral and bilateral aid (Banerji and Anderson 1963), but they went largely silent over the next decades, as the shift from vertical programs to primary health care was advanced and as new multilateral players joined in the effort to improve health. These decades produced other statistical tactics, and new ways of measuring that form a lineage for today's metrics. Among these, was the invention of the QALY, or the quality-adjusted life years metric, by two health economists in 1956.[15]

The QALY was created to determine the value for money of a medical intervention by quantifying the quality of life gained in relation to the cost of that intervention. It allowed planning and policy researchers to "add up" the health benefit in relation to the cost of care, a necessary exercise in an environment of increasingly scarce fiscal resources in the health sector.[16] The popularization of the use of QALYs occurred in the United States and England in ways that shifted not only how health care was figured but also how it was financed. In the United States, where the private sector already played a large role in health care, the QALY helped invigorate evidence-based medicine. Perhaps ironically, although it was designed by economists, the QALY was used to help caregivers and insurers decide how resources should be spent in ways that were based on medical and not simply fiscal priorities.

The impact of QALY thinking was pervasive in the Global North, despite some resistance to evidence-based medicine in the clinic (Timmermans and Berg 2003). More surprising has been how it has trickled out with modifications to the Global South. Economists at the World Bank as early as the 1970s had been interested in health through loans for improved sanitation and the establishment of a Population, Health and Nutrition Department (in 1979), but it was not until the 1990s that the fruition of health policies came into full swing (in the form of structural adjustment policies). These World Bank efforts, in some part, came into direct confrontation with traditional WHO goals (including the provision of essential drugs; Chorev 2012; Keshavjee 2014; Gaudilliere 2015). In taking up the problems of health, World Bank economists were forced to confront the crisis of numbers that plagued health resource decision making in the developing world. That is, a crisis of *funding* produced the QALY in the Global North, but I would argue that it was the crisis of *data* that produced its counterpart, the DALY, in the Global South.

Again, as if repeating the calls for scientific-based evidence in clinical medicine in the Global North (including the establishment of the Cochrane Collaboration; Daly 2005), the call for evidence-based metrics in international health arose at least in part from a perceived lack of accountability in the way health aid had been spent to date but also from recognition that in the developing world, chronic endemic diseases were the norm and yet were not accounted for in mortality statistics. Instead of focusing on incremental gains in quality of life based on treatments, as the QALY does, the team of researchers at the World Bank (Chris Murray, Alan Lopez, and Dean Jamison) invented the DALY as a means to quantify the overall disease burden expressed as number of years lost due to ill health. In essence the DALY provides an economic measure of human productive value by calculating loss of productivity due to disease or disability.

The metrical shift between the QALY and the DALY makes sense since, I would argue, in the Global North what mattered was counting the cost of keeping people alive, whereas in the Global South what mattered was plausible justification for continued expenditures in relation to death *and* disease burdens. These were, in some sense, two sides of the same coin. One focused on mortality (in places where it could plausibly be prevented), and the other focused on life (in places where preventing mortality seemed essentially impossible). The DALY was useful in cost-effectiveness debates and for helping groups like the WHO to determine overall disease burden from specific problems like HIV/AIDS, malaria, and TB on a global scale, which, in turn, justified ongoing health aid investments as problems of global scope. The DALY, in other words, was used to create the most important metric of them all to date: the Global Burden of Disease index, or the GBD.

The actual use of DALYs to get at GBD requires a high level of arithmetic gymnastics to make countries that look nothing like one another metrically comparable. This includes use of social weighting (for age differences: Should disability in a child be counted for the same as that of an adult, and should these be the same across nations?), discounting models (borrowed from economics forecasting to enable valuation of present life in terms of future life years lost, again potentially different between nations), and the use of complex estimates provided by country "experts" for (sometimes contested) data sets on things like actual burden of different disabilities and diseases.

The idea that the DALY created a means of linking health (as a quantified version of the quality of life) to economic models is not surprising. Again, the DALY was originally created for the World Bank and only subsequently used by the WHO to calculate the global burden of disease. Still its creators intended that it would be rolled out on such a large scale that it would "entirely replace traditional approaches to the assessment of health needs as an influence on political decision making" (cited in Arneson and Nord 1999: 1423).[17]

The DALY offers a platform for comparison across national and geographic borders, erasing meddlesome debates about cultural, regional, and national specificities that may have previously made global comparisons impossible or useless (Murray and Lopez 1994a and b). The DALY also solved a perhaps more important problem for policymakers: how to think about allocation of resources in ways that were, in their terms, "value-neutral." One of its chief architects explained this:

> Decision-makers who allocate resources to competing health programmes must choose between the relative importance of different health outcomes such as mortality reduction or disability prevention. Because money is unidimensional, the allocation of resources between programmes defines a set of relative weights for different health outcomes. The only exception to this is in a completely free market for health care where such decisions between competing health programmes are not made by a central authority but by individuals, one health problem at a time. (Murray 1994: 429)

In other words, by assigning numerical values to life and then using complex economic modeling to value that life in relation to productivity, the DALY allowed planners to talk about how to make a situation that does not look like a free-market situation look more like one. That is, the DALY enables us to treat the market as neutral — as a platform for letting the numbers do the work of telling us what works or does not work *as if all else were equal*. But to do so the DALY also has to essentially undertake a "fiscalization" of life. The DALY abstracts quality of life and turns it into a fiscally meaningful form — that is, into an ontological entity that stabilizes messy complexities of "living," that turns life into an object that behaves the way a monetary instrument would behave.

It is not necessarily a bad thing to assign numerical values to expert perception of quality of life. One could think of the DALY and QALY at face value: as exercises in translation between the languages of English and economics, or perhaps as a language that enables a new kind of merger between the World Bank and the WHO.[18] At first glance there is no inherent violence done by the translation. Indeed one could explore the burden of disease as a new technology for the governmentalization of life through the quantification of disability, something that had not previously been possible in relation to policy (Wahlberg and Rose 2015). QALY and DALY metrics enabled planners to not only sidestep politics, but also thorny questions of competing economics platforms and unsolvable debates about structural adjustment vs. charity aid that set the Bank against the WHO. My concern, however, is with what else was accomplished in this move. My concern is with the side effects of the equations; what are we to make of the substitution of a market principle for politics in our thinking about what works in health aid? Because the DALY enables us to track values associated with living (as opposed to dying) in relation to economic modeling, it is worth asking what is at stake when we treat life itself as if it behaved like a monetary instrument — a question that moves in step with but beyond concerns at the WHO over thinking of health in reductionistic economic terms (Chorev 2012).[19] What, in other words, does treating life as a market object do to our thinking about *evidence* in relation to health?

To be sure the DALY's valuing of life in relation to its potential economic productivity is a challenge the DALY architects walk delicately through and around. They acknowledge that it cannot capture the entire range of considerations regarding the value of life or experience of disability. In fact there are several generations of economists who have offered alterations to the model, who have debated the subtleties of weighting for age, gender, national productivity, and so on, and who have questioned its utility altogether.[20] Nevertheless the DALY is still used in health circles far and wide as an instrument for determining how we should be investing our health resources so they are not wasted and for thinking about how our health investments are performing. It continues to be used to justify economic expenditures on health in most countries.

So, despite the weaknesses of the DALY, many global health experts continue to think of it as a success.[21] It continues to generate a certain confidence factor around the data, asserting that even though it is provisional, it is the best we have for knowing what is going on in a form that is neutral by design, not based on politics or ethical bias. In other words, the cleaving to quantitative figuring through the DALY—and the bolstering of its epidemiological platforms in international health work—has been productive, even while being reductive.[22]

The real problem with health economists' use of GBDs and DALYs, it seems, has not really been in the validity of the equation (or whether the equation has got it right) but rather in getting good numbers to fill in the variables in the first place. There is much worry about this, and yet (as Ferguson [1994] notes of development work) this has not stopped anyone from producing lots of them. In fact despite anxieties about inexplicable findings (such as DALYs that show steep declines in TB rates but no drop in new cases; Cohen 2004), the efforts to map GBD through DALYs have not been slowed. The use of them has continued, generating a *lot* of numbers—reams and reams, graphs and graphs, to be exact, forming a cascade of data (pace Basu 2012; Pfeiffer and Chapman 2010).

In the steady and hopeful march toward better accountability in health programs with instruments like the QALY and DALY (and now the newly constructed HALY, or health adjusted life years or even the more abbreviated VLY, value of life years),[23] the emphasis has been on escalating the terms and conditions for data generation. Thus international health workers have recently been tasked with the challenge of finding better and better tools for measuring exactly what is going on when it comes to health and disease and with measuring outcomes to the interventions that are in place. This has been doubly the trend with the emergence of global health, as Gates notes.

In sum, the DALY paved the way for new conversations about how to measure things in global ways, including ways that required a reduction of life to fiscal principles. And just as the QALY generated new conversations about evidence-based medicine in the Global North, the use of DALYs in the Global South has generated parallel conversations about how to do evidence-based global health in ways that are statistically robust yet still useful in our fiscal accounting for outcomes and priorities. But, given the vociferous debates over what the DALYs mean and how hard it is to produce them (and how easy it is to critique them in and around notions of fiscal valuation: the diminishing returns of certainty in debates over how much one life is worth in comparison to another), it is not surprising that Gates believes the search for the new Lord Chancellor is still on. Fortunately he has the chief architect of the DALY, Christopher Murray, on the job.[24]

From Disability-Adjusted Life Years to Experiments

The search for better metrics forms a key ingredient in the reconstitution of international health as "global health." The effort to find better metrics is aided by the fact that economists and clinicians have had to make room for more and more traditional bench and lab scientists who are now (for a variety of clinical, scientific, and market reasons) working on pharmaceutical projects in global places.[25] This inclusion of bench scientists was aided by historic conversations on ensuring essential drugs were affordable (Chorev 2012), the neoliberal legislation and the birth of the World Trade Organization's agreement on trade-related intellection property rights (Gaudilliere 2015), and the rising need among northern scientists for research populations who were drug-naïve (Petryna 2009; Rajan 2006). Along with inclusion of bench bioscientists came the call for new kinds of evidence that would speak the language of not only economists but also bioscientific and pharmaceutical experts. If the DALY was the gold standard for the era of health development, then today the gold standard is a new kind of metric: the statistically robust, randomized and controlled, cost-effectively constituted, experimentally designed, outcome-measurable intervention/research project (or some proximate version thereof).

Again, the history of the randomized controlled trial (RCT) in health care does not begin with global health (Daly 2005). It is also important to remember that the idea RCTs could be of use in improving health care was early on associated with a liberal agenda against conservative economic platforms, even if it was critiqued by some (Lambert 2006; Nichter 2013; Timmermans 2015; Vandenbroucke 2008). Still, the idea that RCT methodologies could be applied to global health and that these methods could solve some of the intractable political debates and problems of evidence have led to its widespread endorsement today, displacing some of the hold that DALYs and QALYs seem to have in institutional settings. Thus, if doing international health in the near past meant participating in a world filled with DALYs, then doing global health today means, more and more, doing *research as intervention* through RCTs, or at least, this is an ideal that is being pushed (Adams 2013a; Erikson 2012).

Long gone are the days of counting simple things like how many vaccines were given out, how many mothers came for prenatal care, or how many babies got oral rehydration solution. DALYs are today often seen as insufficient for the accountability work of global health. Instead, the metrics of choice are RCTs, meaning that interventions must be organized around two kinds of activities: delivering health care and producing usable and reliable data sets that can have a life of their own beyond the intervention. Effective global health work today, in other words, must produce not just health but also statistically robust data that can be powered, subjected to chi-square and linear regressions, and then used for scaling-up. Now, more than ever, we know if we have health only if it can be measured and calculated in these ways. Now, more than ever, we no longer need ministries of health to generate these facts for us (or so we are told) (Rees 2014). All we need is better research designs, controls, randomizations, and sufficient numbers. All we need is more efficient, scientifically minded researchers, and the ability to turn every recipient of health aid into a source of useful metrical data.

The push for use of RCT metrics is indeed widespread. Take a few examples from the *Lancet*'s coverage of the Global Health Metrics and Evaluation Conference, which offers 149 abstracts that demonstrate what can be done with the right tools for measuring. I call attention to the deliberate reference to scientific methods (in italics) in the titles:

"National and Regional Estimates of *Disability-Adjusted Life-Years* (DALYs) in Brazil, 2008: A Systematic Analysis" (Leite et al. 2013)
"Income Shocks and Maternal Health: Evidence from *a Large-Scale Randomised Cash Transfer Experiment* in Zambia" (Peterman et al. 2013)
"Evaluation of a Voucher Programme in Reducing Inequities in Maternal Health Utilisation in Cambodia: *A Quasi-experimental Study*" (Bajracharya et al. 2013)
"What Is a Health Card Worth? *A Randomised Controlled Trial* of an Outpatient Health Insurance Product in Rural India" (Mahal et al. 2013)

"Determining the Cost-Effectiveness of Managing Acute Diarrhea through Social Franchising of ORASEL: *A Randomized Controlled Trial*" (Bishai et al. 2013)

"*Experimental Design*: Impact of an Intervention to Improve Clinic Attendance of Patients with Non-communicable Diseases through Telephone Follow-up" (Hirimuthugoda et al. 2013)

"Risk Factors of Burden of Disease: *A Comparative Assessment* Study for Evidence-based Health Policy Making in Vietnam" (Bui et al. 2013)

"Measuring Local Determinants of Acute Malnutrition in Chad: *A Case-Control Study*" (Tesfai et al. 2013)

Of course, this conference was devoted to the question of metrics and methods, but I believe it suggests the direction in which the standard for doing good global health interventions is moving. Increasingly, doing good global health means setting up one's intervention as a laboratory study in which the ability to get good data—of sufficient quality, sufficient quantity, and demonstrating fidelity of method—matters as much as if not more than the health problem that is being studied. In this conversation the ideal form of intervention is the RCT, but short of that, methods that produce some portion of the RCT, some sort of data that can be used in robust statistical analyses are better than using no statistical metrics at all.

The WHO is on board. In their recent report, "Developing WHO Guidelines with Pragmatic, Structured, Evidence-based Processes" by Chang et al. (2010), they offer a shorthand scaling method for determining the strength of recommendation in relation to the level of evidence provided. The best type of evidence on which to base recommendations, they note, should have "at least one randomized controlled trial with clinical endpoints, or several relevant high quality clinical studies." In the category of "optional" for use in recommendations are the types of evidence-bearing materials that are least reliable: "observational cohort data or at least one case-controlled or analytic study adequately conducted" or (least valuable) "expert opinion based on evaluation of other evidence" (400).

Organizations like the Poverty Action Lab (J-PAL) and Esther Duflo at the Massachusetts Institute for Technology, join this march toward better evidence, suggesting that you can use the RCT method to study the impact of any intervention imaginable, particularly in poverty development work. In the words of its leadership, J-PAL is devoted to training and disseminating the use of RCT methods to study all efforts to reduce poverty (bridging the gap between policy and action in the development field). With a good deal of funding and publication success, the effort to deploy RCT work in the health field has been pursued with parallel enthusiasm. Today, the use of RCTs are encouraged not simply for use in evaluating interventions; they are also meant to be of use in figuring basic health statistics (including those that could be used in formulating DALYs, QALYs, and HALYs).

Anthropologists have been writing about the ethical problems arising from new scientific methods and entanglements of global health (Biehl and Petryna 2013; Crane 2013; Erikson 2012; McGoey et al. 2011; Petryna 2009). Another outcome of the use of scientific metrics is that every kind of health behavior (from latrine use to breastfeeding, use of bed nets, or voucher programs) is now identified as a problem that can be measured in the same way experiments produce data. Experimentally designed global health programs turn complex social behaviors into unilinear variables that perform unproblematically and similarly in statistical models. Like those in curative medicine who tell themselves stories about Aristotelian therapeutics (where all diseases are seen as acute, with a beginning, middle, and end), global health program experts often think they can test effectiveness by creating artificial beginnings, middles, and ends with measurable and definitive outcomes. This tactic also enables us to turn chronic debilitating disorders (like obesity and mental illness) into events that resemble global pandemics requiring urgent attention and measurable intervention outcomes.[26]

The rationale for this reductionism is similar to that used to promote the DALY: it provides what the IHME calls "an impartial, evidence-based picture of global health trends."[27] In other words, the RCT is value-neutral and so does for evidence-based global health scientists what the DALY (and its cost-effectiveness indicators) did for economists. The ideal intervention deploys both: experimental infrastructures of research, preferably incorporating cost-effectiveness as a variable.[28] Like DALYs RCTs have a way of stabilizing some of the background noise that makes one region incomparable with another, one data set useless against another. Ironically, however, RCTs do this not by making global claims but by making local and specific claims that can be scaled up.[29] Thus RCTs become a means of globalizing in slightly different ways than DALYs did by turning our attention to fidelity of research methods so that things can be scaled globally rather than simply getting comparable numbers from region to region, nation to nation. In this way RCTs promote the goal of universal comparability of discrete ontologies of morbidity and mortality but also intervention efficacy, as if these were free-standing global forms of knowledge.

This may be all good, in some sense. It is important to be able to have some measures for knowing what works and what does not work when it comes to global health interventions. It is also important to have reliable methods for comparison that can help inform us about what to do across nations, regions, villages to most effectively bring about health. Still, there are side-effects to the use of these methods that are worth noting. Just as measures like the DALY ran the risk of continually displacing other ways of accounting on grounds that most critics are not qualified to critique the math, so too do those who work in global health feel they must become experts in RCT designs in order to do valid global health work. With the rise in publication of meta-analyses that review previous research on a topic, we find increasingly that what came before the RCT is made to seem as if it did not form an evidence base.[30] The RCT, in other words, makes other ways of accounting for life and health seem soft and unreliable in comparison to the RCT's technical sophistication. How did we ever know anything for sure before the RCT (an interesting question Gates might want to reflect on considering that the RCT was invented nearly a hundred years after the steam engine)?

Similarly, for all of the redemptive euphoria surrounding RCTs, there is a growing sense that the use of RCT metrics is producing both refreshing and troubling effects (similar to but different from those that came with QALYs, DALYs, and HALYs). Anthropologists have been writing against and about the limits of health quantification for some time (Krieger 2012; Lambert 2006; Nichter 2013; Sangaramoorthy and Benton 2012), and there are even health economists who argue that the RCT may not be usable in global health settings (Deaton 2010; Williams 2010).[31] Some researchers are critically exploring the methods of incorporating ethnographic evidence into RCTs as supplemental and also as part of the research design (such as in community participation models of public health) and these accounts show both positive and negative effects (Colvin 2014; Rapkin and Trickett 2005; Smith-Morris, this volume; Smith-Morris et al. 2014).[32] Even with evidence that economics and metrical forms of evidence can sometimes be used to improve health outcomes (such as in tobacco control; Reubi 2013), there are still reasons to be worried.

Already, the requirements for metrics data production have in some global health places created research infrastructures that have become the long-term basis for all transactions in public health. Metrics data collection becomes a passage point through which research teams manage their social relations with study participants, just as such exchanges become the conduit through which health resources are procured (Geissler et al. 2008).[33] These dual purpose relationships can be salutary and they can also be iatrogenic, as when enrolling in clinical trials becomes the only way to gain access to health care (Petryna 2009). Worse, in order for statistically robust research to take place sometimes rural health workers are told to hide evidence, clinicians are inclined to refuse treatment, patients falsify their symptoms to gain enrollment in clinical trials, and clinical infrastructures become undermined by research projects.[34] My own experiences working on safe motherhood in Tibet, where we were told to abandon our project because "not enough women die to get a good power calculation," forms an impetus for this critique and interrogation (Adams 2005, 2013a).[35] The chapters in this volume provide ample evidence of these phenomena.

The more RCT metrics are treated as universally useful, the more they actually create silos of exclusion around what other kinds of evidence, and other methods of creating accountability, are considered valid. Not only do old forms of data collection become suspect, but RCTs can also limit what kinds of things can be done in the world of health intervention simply because the platform for gaining data requires so much, and if these ingredients (these building blocks of the platform) are not available, the interventions often don't get funded. This does not mean that the excluded information is not important in knowing the causes of health, morbidity, and disease or that disorders that cannot be studied are not worth studying. It merely means these nonconforming data, these conditions that cannot be experimentally measured, become invisible to the new funding apparatuses of global health. Meanwhile, the only things that get studied and intervened upon are those that can be measured using RCTs. We might say that in the contemporary global health environment, the RCT may be a new Lord Chancellor.

One could continue down this path, generating fear *not about the failure of the efforts* to do evidence-based global health in this way but rather *about what happens when we succeed in doing so*. Instead of focusing on these down sides, I want to call attention to what else the metrics enable and to the positions and predicaments they put us in in other ways. That is, I am inter-

losing human aspect of medicia

ested in how, even when they fail, these metrics succeed in ways we might be worried about. What I mean by this is that RCT metrics create new conduits for a biopolitical economy, becoming key to the forms of sovereignty that arise with global health and its dreams of health for all. These studies generate forms of success that may even exceed the health benefits that any of these projects claim (Erikson 2012; Harper 2006; Koch 2013). The metrics, that is, return us to certain neoliberal promises, to market opportunities, and ultimately to interventions in sovereignty.[36]

The Win-Win Scenario: Saving Lives and Making Money at the Same Time

interface of capitalism & medicine

Metrics, it seems, allow the transformation of health data into new sources of for-profit capital (see Erikson, this volume). That is, in addition to the fact that technologies of global health pharma and biotech industries work to operationalize neoliberal policies that favor industry goals over the harder-to-measure gains of public health campaigns (Abraham and Ballinger 2012; Rajan 2006), there is another way to think about how metrics, as a form of measurement, are at work in these fiscal adjustments in global health. First, just as the DALY produced a lot of data that had to be managed, the use of these new statistical metrics requires a lot of production technology, and these technologies cost a lot of money. I call attention to a few more of the titles from the *Lancet* special volume on global health (emphasis added):

> "Improving the Usability and Communication of Burden of Disease Methods and Outputs: The Experience of the Burden of Communicable Diseases in Europe *Software Toolkit*" (Cassini et al. 2013)
>
> "Strengthening Vital Registration and Vital Statistics: A Standards-based *Toolkit*" (Horstmann and Lopez 2013)

This talk of toolkits points to the fact that using technological innovation to manage data requires several kinds of productivity: one needs to fix old problems of evidence (getting good data) and also generate new kinds of *products* along the way. The marketing of toolkits and patentable data system programs for running algorithms and managing throughput of large amounts of data has become a new target of opportunity for all of us to do our research, and to potentially profit from it at the same time. The metrics of global health are not simply instruments for the production of evidence; they are profitable products themselves.

The evidence is all around us that we must now innovate to make our research not just cost-recovering and self-sustaining but also profit-generating. The National Science Foundation sent me an email notifying me of a new opportunity for which I was eligible as a former recipient of an NSF award in cultural anthropology. They were offering additional support "in the form of entrepreneurial mentoring, education, and travel funding — to accelerate technology transfer and explore the commercialization of research outcomes." To take advantage of this, I could "write up an executive summary" with a "description of the innovation to be examined for commercialization potential" with "a brief analysis of the potential commercial impact" and "commercialization plan."[37]

We have moved far beyond simple cost-effectiveness here. This linking of health to market concerns is not simply about making sure we distribute health care resources as fairly or equitably as possible. Here we are looking at global health as a market-based profit-driven entrepreneurial opportunity. One can now participate in this entrepreneurial infrastructure that potentially saves lives through profit, and it offers this opportunity by leveraging notions of scientifically derived, objective, evidence-based truth. In other words, the metrics that serve as passage points for good global health work also authorize a new set of linkages between market-based problem solving and global health targets.

The shifts in global health toward gaining an upper hand on accountability are *not necessarily* designed with neoliberal outcomes in mind. But there have been underlying transformations in how we all think about what counts as evidence and how we are going to pay for the costly endeavor of taking care of those who are not healthy and cannot pay for themselves, for their health care infrastructures, or for doing research. How we think about what constitutes good evidence has direct implications for the sorts of economic practices of globalization that structure global health. In this sense the embrace of market-sensitive techniques that are tied to irreducible forms of metrics accountability works seamlessly with the political aspirations of neoliberal reforms. The notion that we all need to use better metrics is authorized by claims to scientific objectivity and rigor, and it also happens to enable us to think that making profits on the patenting and commercializing of products for doing this sort of work is simultaneously a good thing for health (McGoey et al. 2011). Here the scientific metrics indirectly become the micropractices of neoliberalism.

It is useful to recall that the invention of "global health" was itself not simply a call for more global perspectives or solutions than had been seen previously. It was adopted, at least in part, in 1992 by the WHO in response to aggressive new incursions of the World Bank, UNICEF (the Global Fund), the Rockefeller Foundation, and the Gates Foundation into international health governance (Brown et al. 2006; Crane 2013: 152).[38] That is, global health was not only a political turf war; it was also a response to the ever-increasing incursions of market- and private-sector logics in the postwar state-funded architecture of organizations like the WHO.[39] This, in and of itself, may be a reflection of the larger role played by economists in the policymaking of global health since the 1990s (via the World Bank in particular; Chorev 2012).

This trend toward leveraging the market and its fiscal opportunities by putting them to work in health may have begun back with the DALY and QALY. In Britain the QALY helped the public organization that sponsored its use to leave its home under the British Health Authority and become a private company (Banerjee, Hollis, and Pogge's 2013 Health Impact Fund, which Erikson writes about, this volume) that Bloomberg pays a good deal of attention to, not just because it is a publicly traded company but because it uses the QALY to rate various medical technologies, drugs, and procedures that are coming onto the medical marketplace. In this model the government pays out (in the same way it does with social impact bonds) profits to companies that have invested in health. That is, if health improves, the bonds pay off. In global health, there are similar trends as the lion's share of funding for global health shifts from government-sponsored multilateral agencies to private foundations, but in global health it is not entirely clear what equations between "success," health, and profits are in play. What is clear is that metrics are the key to their use at all.

So, for instance, the Global Fund and the Gates Foundation offer two interesting models for how to privatize and put the market to work for global health. Before we turn to their use of metrics, it is worth noting that the shift to private wealth philanthropy to fill in where public institutions have lost public funding for their work has come about mostly because of good intentions. Still, this shift has arguably conferred on people like Bill and Melinda Gates the privileges once reserved for nobility or heads of state when it comes to standard-setting agendas, even when they surround themselves with experts from the field.[40] Small and local NGOs often feel at the mercy of capriciousness and instability tied to subtle shifts in the changing priorities of mega-donors. The powerful donor-driven agendas of the new players in global health also come with a surprisingly optimistic rhetoric about problem solving even while sometimes reinventing old and worn wheels from an era of international health or even an era of colonial medicine (Birn 2005, 2014). Some are noting how privately funded alliances between public institutions and private philanthropy complicate traditional analytical categories between markets and states, publics and privates, society and capitalism, blurring them in ways that are both exciting and troubling (Adams 2013b; Craddock 2012). But, this blurring can also fuel more traditional market opportunities and arrangements. That the Gates Foundation invests in global health solutions that are tethered inextricably to the industries hoping to make profits on these interventions (in pharmaceuticals and technologies; Erikson this volume) might be a win-win scenario. But the lack of a firewall between profit opportunities and health rights can also authorize subtle shifts in profit-seeking away from health and toward stock index bottom lines, especially when cost-effectiveness is a variable in the study. Should we be frightened to learn, for instance, that the creation of new Global Health Investment Fund (with JPMorgan Chase and Co.) and many other spin-off ventures for global health have made global health one of the fastest growing opportunities for the *for-profit* world of investing (again, as Erikson, this volume)? Or should this be celebrated? Should we be worried that some of these funds earn profits from industries implicated in causal ways in the high rates of disease and disability in countries where the Global Health Fund wants to improve health outcomes? Or, is this a necessary evil in a pragmatic arrangement that otherwise works well?

Advocates of private and public-private alliances argue that it is a good thing to get profit-driven industries (and Wall Street institutions) involved in global health. That is where the money is, therefore where the funders are these days, and private sector funding liberates global health programs from cumbersome demands of bilateral and multilateral political institutions (not to mention regulations; Craddock 2012). Still, just how these public-private infrastructures measure health outcomes alongside fiscal profits is not entirely transparent.

In public-private partnerships like the Health Impact Fund (tied to the QALY, above) governments are asked to pay investors profits if and only if health targets are met; there are no similar guarantees in the fully private model. In the Global Health Investment Fund, for instance, it appears that investments from JP Morgan Chase (and other investors) provide the operating capital for developing health-products (technologies, pharmaceuticals), but returns for its investors are not necessarily directly tied to health outcomes. If I understand it correctly, the fund grows by generating the right kind of data, the right kind of metrics that show profits *can* be made on things that promise to improve health (vaccines, clean water technologies, etc.). Interestingly, this means that investors can potentially reap rewards from the fund just by showing that an intervention or product is scalable. Knowing what is scalable means having the kinds of metrics that show this. Whether or not the product is implemented, how one might measure the health impact from it, and what was lost in the production of this kind of knowledge are not outcomes necessary for the fund to earn money. In other words, what enables these calculations of profit to be made at every step of the way is the metrics (and particularly RCTs). RCTs show the investment potential of technologies and interventions *by showing they can be scaled up*. With good data the fund can get up and running. Again, how one counts *health* as a result of these investments, is no longer essential to profitmaking. Profit can be made entirely on the promise of scaling up.

The Global Fund, for its part, shows similar trends toward privatization and toward the use of metrical indices of outcome that have as much to do with fiscal as with health returns. In fact the Global Fund was a public-private partnership formed around the urgent need to create funding streams for AIDS, TB, and malaria (and received large contributions from Gates Foundation, Credit Suisse, and the superpowers). In diverting funds from existing bilateral and multilateral agencies and putting them into the hands of a new regime of experts (including Jeffry Sachs and Richard Feacham), the Global Fund called attention to its key intervention: not doing "business as usual" but rather holding itself to "new levels of fiscal accountability."[41] In a nutshell the goal was to create new ways of evaluating not simply "what money was spent on" but also on "what targets had been achieved." Laudable goals that ostensibly included health outcomes as measures of success. But, to do this work, the fund also created "co-branded indexes that could be licensed as the basis for investment products." In other words, the strategy for earning profits was on the indices, not necessarily on health outcomes.

The Global Fund, originally modeled as a unit of the UN and housed therein, was in fact set up to leverage private sources of wealth capital — again, a strategy that was in some sense unavoidable given the fact that the largest pots of money available for things like this were held by these private entities. Large pharmaceutical companies were also brought to the table, and while they were asked to eliminate profiteering on things like HIV cocktails, they were also invited to participate in the capitalization opportunities of global health in new ways (Cooper 2008). In the Global Fund, however, the mergers went beyond pharmaceutical interests and far beyond simply leveraging private and corporate wealth for the work of publicly oriented global health. The mergers and the commitments to market-driven solutions have impacted the very business of how we think of doing global health work as a product-oriented marketable set of practices. S&P Dow Jones Indices (a leading investment company) signed on to explore the creation of cobranded indexes with the Global Fund in 2010. Metrics, and the creation of brandable toolkit strategies for measuring health intervention outcomes on a global scale, have again become a profit-making endeavor while creating opportunities for the project of global health to "pay for itself."[42] When making profits on health investments is part of the modus operandi of the institution, the question of how and when profits become as important, if not more important, than health needs to be vigilantly kept on the table.

Again, absolutely key to the rise in this version of the public-private partnership is the notion that we will be able to rigorously show outcomes that justify the delivery of profits on these technologies and interventions.[43] Without agreed-upon metrics that can generate the evidence of success or failure, these partnerships cannot work.[44] The RCT provides one such metric, and its malleability as an instrument for measuring possibility (and not just health effects) in promises of scaling up is a key to its use in this global health economy.

This becomes more and more visible in new technology companies that hope to build businesses around appropriate technologies for use in global health efforts. A company called Vestergaard (formerly with Frandsen), for instance, works on developing technologies and implementation programs for diarrhea, malaria, and HIV in Africa. (One of their technologies is the LifeStraw, now being explored by Peter Redfield.) According to one of their representatives (as presented at GHECon at UCSF Global Health Sciences in 2013), the company abides by the logic that "if you can't scale it up, don't do it." So, what enables companies like this to exist is the idea that one can get statistically significant measurable impacts (using evidence-based techniques) that show outcomes, thereby enabling the sort of scale-up that will justify the profits that the partner (for-profit) companies hope to accrue. How metrics are able to show scalability, however, depends on what kind of outcomes are included. Scalability should be measured in relation to a reduction in water-borne diseases, for instance, not just in relation to the distribution and use of the technologies. International health old-timers who recall the trials and tribulations of ensuring correct technology use (of everything from condoms to antibiotics) might take peculiar interest in how technologies like these will be able to avoid the messy and complicated (and woefully impossible to study using RCTs) realities of implementation, let alone health outcomes. The question of choice of metrics to use in these exercises in accountability thus migrate to the forefront of debates over whether or not this medical experiment of mixing profits with health will work at all. But, it is clear that profitability may not depend on that sort of calculation at all.

end goal of impact

As RCT strategies tie us to the terms of reference used by investment bankers, providing us with the rationale for investing more money and time as measured in "scalability," are we in and through RCT metrics simultaneously asked to think about health as if it were also measurable in these terms? Here is the logical next step in the fiscalization of life. Instead of quantifying the quality of life to justify fiscal interventions in health, we now justify profit opportunities in and through a metricization process that subordinates life to its role in intervention/investment opportunities. Life (or better said, disease and infirmity) is merely a passage point on the way to getting the numbers that will let the market grow.

The truth is, good numbers are hard to get, and sometimes they have to be forged out of imperfect numbers and sometimes they have to hide the fact that they lie. As the terms and conditions of evidence are increasingly tied to RCTs, however, so too are the only empirical claims that are brought to the table those that can be generated using an RCT design. These scenarios offer further evidence that RCT metrics are the new Lord Chancellor.[45] This type of arrangement goes far beyond the mere profiting of pharmaceutical companies in the global health world (Cooper 2008; Rajan 2006) by transforming any and potentially all interventions into for-profit possibilities by way of RCTs. The new metrics create promissory futures in which only interventions that work or promise product lines through scale-up are deployed, diseases are eradicated more swiftly and treated more effectively by these simple techniques of production and counting, and money is not just saved but also produced along with (by way of) the project of saving lives.[46]

It may be win-win sometimes, but I would add that regardless of how one feels about the potential successes or failures of profit-seeking models of global health (or about the potential moral corruptions of profit), the real problem is slightly different. There is a very fine line between *using RCTs to do the sort of health work we want to do and doing only the sort of work that RCTs can be designed to do.* We are taught to think that RCT numbers will in some sense do the work of thinking for us by giving us numbers, and that these numbers will be powerful neutral tools for policymaking and for intervention itself. But using RCTs is also teaching us to think always about how to get the numbers to show that one intervention is better than another, and if we can't find these numbers we run the risk of not doing these projects at all, underline even when we know they work.

With the imperative for data-driven research being what it is, and the ways in which investments in global health are orchestrated around win-win opportunities for fiscal rewards alongside (sometimes perhaps even without health rewards), it is not surprising to learn of a recent World Bank Blog post that calls for ending the problem of "data deprivation." The authors write,

> About half the countries we studied in our recent paper, "Data Deprivation, Another Deprivation to End," are deprived of adequate data on poverty. This is a huge problem because the poor, who often lack political representation and agency, will remain invisible unless objective and properly sampled surveys reveal where they are, and how they're faring. The lack of data on human and social development should be seen as a form of deprivation, and along with poverty, *data deprivation* should be eradicated.[47]

Given the current models for funding and the imperatives for generating evidence that can be used in metrics calculations for health investments, it makes sense to think of some people as having a crisis of "data deprivation." The blog authors may be right. These days, lacking data may be even more tragic than lacking health.

Governance and the Empire of Data

Metrics today allow new global health commitments to public-private partnerships that, in turn, allow private-sector profit concerns to serve as the index makers for our excursions into the worlds of counting and creating health.[48] They also radically alter the terms and conditions for receiving funds from donor agencies and for justifying expenditures in money-making opportunities in global health. Instead of funding being based solely on demonstrations of neediness, today RCTs enable donors to base funding decisions on evidence that things *are* working, even if this also means producing profits for investors by not funding those interventions that cannot produce this evidence (again, even if we know they work). I argue that this predicament returns us, finally, to questions of sovereignty.[49]

"Life," known in and through the experiment and its metrical accountability, has become fertile ground for the circulations of capital and, I would add, the exercises of sovereignty that come with it. Sovereignty here is subordinated to the operations of capital that are transacted in and through a borderless, biological, postcrisis, but still medically needy humanity. We have known for some time that universalized tactics of statistics and counting work as much as performative instruments are methodological tactics of the empirical, and that these have been implicated in both colonial and postcolonial strategies of governance (Geltzer 2009; Shore and Wright 2015; Silverstein 2014). Less clearly articulated is how performative metrics like the RCT authorize bypassing the nation-state while suturing economic opportunities to the work of global public health and its large public-private partnerships.

Following Achille Mbembe's (2001) careful analysis of the demise of the territorial state in the postcolony and Michael Hardt and Antonio Negri's (2001) proposition that sovereignty is best apprehended in terms of empire, I would argue that these metric practices ultimately invite us to come to terms with a new kind of "global sovereign." This sovereign is a flexible assemblage of data production, number crunching, and scale-up profit sourcing that, like Mbembe's fetish, orchestrates biopolitical health interventions so that they work within capitalism's terms and limits and so that they serve the global architecture of neoliberal debt and profit economies. These metrics are flexible and demanding, adjustable to local conditions yet inclined to answer to one master; above all, these metrics make it easy to reduce complex problems of health to problems of counting and creating research platforms, whether or not they ever actually improve health in the places where they are set in motion.

In and through the metric machineries of global health that turn intervention into a potentially money-producing, capital-investing, resource-generating opportunity, regimes of counting interrupt and often replace traditional practices of governance in sovereign nations, guiding decision making about health investments and accountability. For all that these metrics do to make it easy to reduce complex problems of health to problems of counting and creating research platforms, it is not clear yet that they actually improve health in any of the places where they are used. In some cases, the metrics become a technology of death as much as of life.[50]

Finally, insofar as the notion of "the global" that is at work in these institutions is one that hopes, rather deliberately, to transcend the nation-state (and all of its flaws; Rees 2014), this outcome seems unsurprising. The challenges of how states navigate a politics of life and death through these metrics and these new alliances of industry and health (even those which recognize some sense of national involvement)[51] become, in turn, more significant than ever.

Database Determinism and Its Residual Stories

Don Brenneis (2010) borrows the phrase *database determinism* to describe how number-crunching metrics are being used to determine and assess quality of productivity in the academy. The problem with having data sets, he notes, is that they ultimately compel a kind of utility that might not otherwise be seen. Audit cultures abide by the principle "If you've got it, use it." I think those of us working in global health feel at times pulled in by the inertia of certainty and fungibility that is created in the wake of metrics-driven database determinism. At the same time, I would argue that just as the reductionist metrics of the QALY and DALY tended to create eddies of omission in their wake — always the search for better numbers — so too do the metric instruments associated with experimental platforms and RCTs produce residuals that cannot be contained by the metrics. That is, there seems to always be a "surfeit" in these metrics — the things that slip out of numerical grasp, formed in the wake of the large-scale rolling out of these tools. It is the production of these excesses, alongside its profits, that I have pointed to in this essay.

Set against or seen as incomprehensible in the world of RCTs one finds a persistence of older forms of knowledge and rhetorical practices that historically have been used in the transactions of health aid. George Weisz (2005) refers to this as the pathos (affect) that works sometimes with and sometimes against the logos (evidence) generated by experience in the clinical setting. In global health pathos arises in the form of the compelling case study, the moving story, and the anecdote, all of which are positioned as alternative forms of evidence in statistics-oriented RCT global health. These forms of narrative, image, and affect have always been related in complex ways to practices of counting in health (even during colonial eras), but I would argue that today these forms of knowledge become encased as a kind of new residual in global health work precisely because of the ways our contemporary metrics practices push them out of the epistemological frame of evidence-based medicine. I would argue that they are residual, however, in the sense that they form a surplus that is recuperated in an affective play to affirm the numbers.

Small- and large-scale NGOs, for example, are notoriously good at using the trope of what Butt (2002) has called accounts of "the suffering stranger" to raise funds. But the use of suffering stranger stories is as common in multimillion-dollar aid charities like Save the Children Fund as it is in smaller, politically engaged organizations like the one I worked with, called One HEART. Every few months I get a postcard or letter from One HEART sharing the personal story of a woman or child who has been given "life" because of the daring and committed work of One HEART but, more important, from the support it has received from people like me.

The annual reports of large global health NGOs are full of these accounts. Melinda Gates, in her portion of the foundation's annual letter, offers the moving story of meeting Sadi Seyni in Niger. A young mother who had given birth to five children, she didn't learn about contraceptives until after her second child. Sadi wants more children but now knows that getting a contraception injection is healthier for her and her children because she can space her pregnancies. Melinda Gates writes, "Every time I come back from a trip, I am overflowing with stories about why women like Sadi are so inspiring to me" (M. Gates 2013).

Even the global health textbooks that argue for the rigorous use of statistical metrics offer vivid and gripping stories: Laurie Smith, living in Portsmouth, Virginia, who comes down with meningitis from West Nile virus; Getachew, a twenty-year-old Ethiopian with HIV; Jim Smith, a high school student in London who has TB. The story of Shawki, a sixty-year-old Jordanian living in Amman, prompts us to ask questions about how we can know, for sure, what led to his diabetes. Is it his poverty, his wealth, his genetics? The authors who present these people to us assure us that studies that use reliable methods like those of evidence-based RCT (or RCT-like) research will tell us the answers to their questions (Merson et al. 2012; Skolnick 2012).

This skillful manufacture of stories offers more than local color to the real work of a global health scientist who ultimately knows that it doesn't matter what their names are or where they are from; what matters is what the numbers tell us as truths about their situations. However, I would argue that these stories do much more than reveal how diseases are global and how global health is not simply for the global poor in out-of-the-way places relative to the industrialized North. These stories do the heavy lifting of creating a basis for legitimacy and authority that the numbers cannot provide.[52]

importance of a narrative

We might benefit from a venture into making sense of the way these two kinds of evidence are asked to dance — perhaps in a tango — in the world of global health, but at the outset I would argue that the circulation of story evidence is not uncommon because it holds affective power. Stories carry a different kind of credibility because they make people feel something quite different from what they feel when they see compelling numbers. That is, stories may tap into the same sense of urgency, but they arouse a different sentiment of attachment and compassion than numbers do. I would say that it is this surfeit of emotional connection it arouses that makes the work not only morally compelling but also believable as a human endeavor that hopes for efficacy.

Affective evidence forms a spectral possibility, perpetuating a fantasy of intimacy and social responsibility on which relations of care and sensibilities of obligation rest. This evidence often includes vivid representations of a kind of obscenity of poverty's violence. The narrative story thus has a productive relationship with metrics. *By being ostensibly excluded from the regimes of truth making that are tied to mathematical figuring, stories are left to carry a nonneutral moral certainty that mathematics and RCTs claim deliberately and victoriously to avoid but are, in fact, haunted by as a spectral display that they need.*

That is, it may be that metrics create the space for certainty in forms of truth-telling that, in the end, exceed the metrics themselves. Stories do a lot of the work of "efficacy productivity" when it comes to funding and to convincing everyone who does not speak math (and perhaps even those who do) of the worthiness of various interventions. Like residuals in market transactions, these stories generate a symbolic capital that is reinvested in order to fuel the industries of number crunching in important new ways. What is certain about the new metrics, however, is that no matter what economists, epidemiologists, or even anthropologists hope for them, they are indelibly marked as political, they are never really neutral, and they are almost always quite messy. It is perhaps for this reason that having great stories to back them up seems to give them a kind of credibility that, left to their own devices, the raw numbers never really seem to offer.

So where does this leave us, and what possibility is there that these stories might do the opposite (as promised in the work of many anthropologists today)? What is the chance that stories might not just serve the metrics but actually discredit them or force them to be reconsidered? In the end I believe that while stories in and of themselves do not usually possess the epistemological weight needed to undo the methodological certainty of numbers—that is, they seldom create space for rethinking what we mean by evidence and by metrics or how to undo them (or at least they seldom do this in the right crowds, times, and places)—I remain hopeful that it is in this space that is often left unattended by the numbers, this space of storytelling where (even while being sutured to the numbers), one might find holes in the sovereign forms that (directly and indirectly) aspire to govern in our global times.

Notes

Thanks to audiences at the conference: From International to Global: Knowledge, Diseases and the Postwar Government of Health, an international conference sponsored by DRC, Cermes, Inserm, and CNRS, Paris France, Feb 12–14, McGill University, Social Studies of Medicine (particularly Tobias Rees, Margaret Lock, Pierre Minn, and Fiona Gedeon Achi); Duke Global Health Institute (and Harris Solomon); Princeton University Global Health Colloquium (particularly Joao Biehl and students), the ISSI Seminar series at UC Berkeley, as well as audiences in the Global Health Group at UC Davis and in the Medical Anthropology Speakers Series at Stanford University.

1. "Is Paris Worth a Mass?," *Economist*, January 12, 2013, 14.

2. Porter (1992) reminds us that although the mathematical techniques existed much earlier in the nineteenth century, the scientific project of using these techniques to talk about societies took much more work. It required transforming mathematical techniques for predicting error into a set of positive instruments that would create singular truths from large and diverse numbers: "The regularity of crime, suicide, and marriage

when considered in the mass was invoked repeatedly to justify the application of statistical methods to problems in biology, physics and economics" (6).

3. The sciences of society, including those focused on health, family life, and ritual behaviors, were adjunct to the sciences that used numerics, from economics to statistics, that were used in colonial enterprises. For specific historians, see the introduction, this volume.

4. There is a much longer story about the ways that humanitarianism and health development have become friends, enemies, and friends again (Chandler 2001). The gradual merging of such "rights" discourse with that of "needs-based" interventions paved the way for an eventual blurring of development aid programs and those of NGO humanitarian groups and a renewed commitment to taking political sides.

5. The pitfalls of the back and forth on neoliberal policies, and the pitfalls of neoliberal policy *success* in international health efforts to control TB, are well captured by Keshavjee (2014).

6. The MDGs were rolled out originally in 2000 but modified and updated annually with insights from the UN Open Working Group's Sustainable Development Goals (SDG) report (Buse and Hawkes 2015).

7. The editorial essay by Katz (2008) offers a good example of the critique, along with the collected works of Paul Farmer. My discussion of political will here is in reference to the problems Chorev (2012) identifies in relation to the nation-state (also described in the introduction).

8. This version of finding a solution that is "above" politics is also found in mission statements of humanitarian health aid groups like Medecins Sans Frontiers, discussed at more length by Redfield (2013).

9. Evidence for this is also found in a Gates Foundation report by Suprotik Basu, who writes, "The single most important thing we must do if we hope to achieve the Health [Millennium Development Goals] is to sharpen our focus on monitoring and reporting—and specifically, to embrace imperfect data." His logic is that numbers are vital, thus use of imperfect numbers is better than no use of numbers at all. Suprotik Basu, "Even Imperfect Data Can Save Lives," Bill and Melinda Gates Foundation, September 9, 2013, accessed December 18, 2013, http://www.impatientoptimists.org/Posts/2013/09/Progress-on-MDGs-Requires-an-Obsession-for-Tracking-Results.

10. Petryna (2009), Biehl (2008, 2013), and Crane (2013) discuss global health in terms of the ethics of ownership, authority, and partnership in the coproduction of scientific knowledge in peripheral locales.

11. Rees (2014) proposes that this aspiration might itself instantiate a new form of governance based on a global, post–nation-state notion of biological humanity. Haskell (1985) provides an excellent overview of the optimism found at the core of Gates's hopes to marry private-sector resources to public problems and solve them by using better science (in this case metrics). He writes, "Among all the new techniques that flourished under the encouragement of the market, none did more to stretch people's sense of personal power—and therefore to extend their sense of causal involvement in other lives—than contractualism itself. And among all the sources of the humanitarian sensibility, none was more important than the contribution made by a promise-keeping

form of life: a heightened sense of personal effectiveness created by the possession and use of powerful recipes—recipes made powerful in part by the growing calculability of a market society that tethered each ego to its own past intentions with 'long chains of will,' even as this society liberated each ego from traditional constraints on personal ambition" (1985: 559).

12. *Lancet* 377 (9770), 2011.

13. This emerges even earlier, as Erikson (2012: 371) notes when, in 2005, *Lancet* editors began to call for better statistics for evaluating health interventions and outcomes.

14. A story well told by Rees (2014).

15. Christopher Cundell and Carlos McCartney. See "Quality-Adjusted Life Year," Blogspot, January 30, 2011, accessed January 20, 2014, http://qualityadjusted1.blogspot .com/2011/01/debate.html.

16. The QALY offered a way to make population-level comparisons between people with similar and different disorders, thus helpful for health planning and spending at the national level.

17. Taken from the "International Burden of Disease Network. Report of the foundation meeting. Atlanta: International Burden of Disease Network; 1998," as cited in Arneson and Nord 1999.

18. See Pfeiffer and Chapman (2010) on impacts of structural adjustment policies that preceded the development of the DALY, and the relationships between the WHO and the World Bank that led to the latter's eventually superseding the former. The World Bank's production of its "World Development Report 1993: Investing in Health" (led by Chris Murray and Dean Jamison, with Murray going on to develop the GBD instruments) is a turning point for this interest on the part of the Bank in health matters. Chorev (2012: 150) describes the *Lancet* editorial that attests to how this report marks the shift in leadership on international health from the WHO to the World Bank.

19. How it does this is not entirely obvious. Murray (1994: 435) notes that "because the human capital approach inadequately reflects human welfare, productivity weights are *not used* in the development of DALYs." Instead the DALY uses a notion of "social roles," which still, not surprisingly, weight more heavily losses to disability that occur in the middle age range rather than at the beginning or end of the life course.

20. The major critic of the GBD approach (Williams 1999) pointed out the weakness of measuring disability against interventions, of allowing value (as a form of bias) in determining life expectancy, as well as weighting practices in relation to questions of quality of life, and more. These of course also provoked responses (Murray and Lopez 1996, 2000). Among the many concerns were that it presupposed that life years of disabled people were worth less than life years of people without disabilities; that it did not take into account comorbidities; that age weighting disfavors children and the elderly; that life estimates disfavor women; that it reflects values of societal usefulness rather than individual utility of life (Anand and Hanson 1997; Arnesen and Nord 1999; Gold et al. 2002).

21. On clinical rejection of evidence-based forms of knowledge, see Lambert 2006; Timmermans and Berg 2003; Waitzkin 2011. On the history of counting in Western clinical medicine, see Navarro 1978; Waitzkin 2011; Weisz 2005.

22. See the report by Arnesen and Kapiriri (2004) that discusses the ways value-laden assumptions change priorities for health planning in countries.

23. The HALY is a combined measure, including morbidity and mortality impact on life years, the VLY "value of life years" measure is useful to economists who, for instance, in the Global Health 2035 manifesto (Jamison et al. 2015), want to quantify the return on investment in health for middle-income countries.

24. Christopher Murray, who was trained as both a PhD in health economics and an MD, is now at the Institute on Health Evaluation and Metrics, which is largely funded by the Bill and Melinda Gates Foundation and operates as a public private partnership with the University of Washington.

25. This is in part because of big pharma's need for drug-naïve research subjects and in part because of the market forces behind global health (that Craddock, this volume, identifies).

26. Some researchers also talk about the need to use models rather than RCTs for measuring effectiveness of impacts. However, most of these studies that veer away from the use of rigid RCT designs still use cost-effectiveness as a means of creating metric uniformity.

27. "History," Institute for Health Metrics and Evaluation, accessed July 10, 2013, http://www.healthmetricsandevaluation.org/about-ihme/history. Reaccessed at http://www.healthdata.org/about/history, May 28, 2015.

28. See the work at the Poverty Action Lab and the work of Duflo et al. (2008).

29. Thanks to Fiona Gendeon Achi at McGill University for pointing this out to me.

30. This process replicates the early history of the use of evidence-based medicine in public health, exemplified by the Cochrane Collaboration (Daly 2005).

31. Deaton (2010) argues that RCTs often cannot account for heterogeneity or exogeneity the way they are used in global health settings.

32. Incorporating qualitative information in systematic ways into large-scale health planning exercises, even at the WHO (Colvin 2014), duplicates previous iterations of such efforts beginning in the 1970s and are equally fraught. Mandates for fidelity often erase the specificities that qualitative methods produce and that explain program success or failure (see Smith-Morris, this volume).

33. See also the work of Ashley Ouvrier.

34. This work follows a long list of scholars who have been exploring these things: Allotey et al. 2003; Becker et al. 2013; Crane 2013; Erikson 2012; Janes and Chuluundorj 2004; Nichter 2008; Petryna 2009; Pfeiffer 2004; Pfeiffer and Chapman 2010. For accounts of positive impacts of health research infrastructures, see Reynolds Whyte (2014).

35. There are exceptions to the trend. In public health, for example, see Holmes 2013; Pisani 2009.

36. Scholars who are writing about the limitations of RCT work in implementation efforts of behavioral prevention sciences include Rapkin and Trickett 2005; Deaton 2010.

37. The site information changes regularly. The homepage for the site which was

sent to me in an email is: NSF I-Corps Contact, http://www.nsf.gov/news/special
_reports/i-corps. National Science Foundation, "Innovation Corps Teams Program
(I-Corps Teams): Program Solicitation." It contained these suggestions when accessed
June 28, 2013, http://www.nsf.gov/pubs/2012/nsf12602/nsf12602.pdf.

38. Brown et al. (2006) state that it was not "invented" by the WHO, but their article
maps out how, in fact, the WHO was the major player to consolidate the movement.

39. This is in addition to the shift toward biosecurity (Lakoff 2010), and Cooper
(2008) and McGoey et al. (2011) note the shift toward pharmaceuticalization.

40. See McCoy et al.'s (2009) critical review of Gates Foundation funding priorities:
(1) selection of funding priorities (based on personal networks and relationships rather
than anonymous peer review); (2) promotion of privatized health care provision in
low- and middle-income countries (and helping the World Bank advance these priorities without clear evidence that private-sector solutions work better); (3) challenges
to multilateral global health governance structures and policymaking; (4) prioritizing
technological and pharmaceutical solutions over other kinds of solutions (a bias that
is consistent with Gates's own business successes but not one that is necessarily shown
to work in international health); (5) questions about prioritization of diseases based
on these technological and pharmaceutical resources rather than on evidence of need
in the countries where it works (although this may be a strategy aimed at filling gaps in
existing resource provision (see Birn 2005). They write, "In view of its receipt of public
subsidies in the form of tax exemptions, there should be an expectation that the foundation is subject to some public scrutiny" (1652). A *Lancet* editorial (2009: 1577) also
points to risk of the growing monopoly of the Gates Foundation.

41. See Horton 2013; Commission on Macroeconomics and Growth, "Investment in
Global Health Will Save 8 Million Lives a Year and Generate at Least a $360 Billion An-
nual Gain within 15 Years, Says a New Report Presented to WHO," press release, December 20, 2001, accessed June 28, 2013. http://en.wikipedia.org/wiki/The_Global_Fund
_to_Fight_AIDS,_Tuberculosis_and_Malaria.

42. S&P Dow Jones Indices, "The Global Fund Fight AIDS, Tuberculosis and Malaria,
Dow Jones Indexes Sign Memorandum to Explore Creation of Co-Branded Indexes,"
press release, March 4, 2010, accessed July 30, 2013. http://press.djindexes.com/index
.php/the-global-fund-to-fight-aids-tuberculosis-malaria-dow-jones-indexes-sign
-memorandum-to-explore-creation-of-co-branded-indexes/.

43. We might look at the Social Impact Bond strategies as falling into this camp as
well. See Ian Galloway, "Pay for Success Financing," *Federal Reserve Bank of San Francisco* 9(1), 2013. These are a way of incentivizing businesses to get more involved in the
work of financing the safety net for a profit. The private sector funds the bonds for the
charity work, and if they show success, the government pays them back with interest.

44. The work on evidence-based advocacy by Storeng and Behague (2014) is particularly clear on this, and also on the pitfalls of this approach.

45. One frequently hears global health experts saying they expect a return on investment and that they cannot "do research for research's sake." Basu (2011) points to
the revolving door between philanthropic organizations and corporate board member-

ship for companies that will benefit from the programs that are funded by the philanthropies, sidestepping thorny problems of conflict of interest. Erikson (this volume) takes up these linkages in detail.

46. On the upside of this alliance, see Craddock (2012). For the downside, see Parker and Allen (2014). I also recall the useful history of scalability by Tsing (2012), who traces its roots to colonialism and capitalism and offers a useful critique by focusing on the virtues and dangers of nonscalability.

47. Serajuddin et al., 2015, accessed May 29, 2015, http://blogs.worldbank.org /developmenttalk/much-world-deprived-poverty-data-let-s-fix.

48. A possibility that must repeat at every step the onerous burden of recognizing that "if it can't be enumerated, it won't work" (Erikson 2012: 381).

49. See Biruk (2012) for an example of the links between health development research and the state in Malawi.

50. Mbembe's (2001: 23) insight that Carl Schmitt's "definition of sovereignty at the beginning of the twentieth century, namely, the power to decide on the state of exception" at the dawn of the postcolony is useful here, for it is the acts of both making visible and making invisible (deciding which deaths count and which will not) that have become key ingredients in the global health apparatuses of statecraft in many places today.

51. As is called for in the Global Health 2035, or the "Grand Convergence" effort in grand global health planning (Jamison et al., 2015).

52. I am reminded by a reviewer that it is possible to talk about how these stories produce other outcomes as well, including xenophobia and violence. These too can work to bolster intervention prospects.

PART I. GETTING GOOD NUMBERS

2 · ESTIMATING DEATH A Close Reading of Maternal

Mortality Metrics in Malawi CLAIRE L. WENDLAND

Two Conversations

In 2010 a debate broke out over exactly how bad maternal mortality was worldwide. It was clear to epidemiologists and policymakers that the fifth Millennium Development Goal—to reduce maternal mortality by three quarters between 1990 and 2015—would not be met. Where there was no consensus, however, was just how far off the world would be.

Two important papers provided two different answers. In the *Lancet* researchers from the University of Washington's Institute for Health Metrics and Evaluation (IHME) claimed a small but steady drop in maternal deaths worldwide, based on measures from 181 countries over the period 1980–2008 (Hogan et al. 2010). The authors calculated that death rates would have dropped more substantially in the absence of the HIV pandemic. Even with HIV, however, they calculated that things had improved, if slowly and slightly, for mothers worldwide.

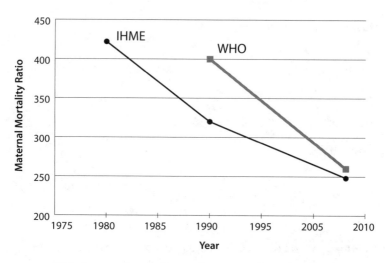

FIGURE 2.1 · Global maternal mortality trends: IHME and WHO estimates.

Sources: Hogan et al. 2010; World Health Organization 2010.

An editorial accompanying the *Lancet* paper celebrated the good news as "robust reason for optimism" after two decades of little improvement in maternal health: the editorialist described this prolonged lack of progress as "one of the most deforming scars on the body of global health" (Horton 2010: 1581).

Five months later a collaborative group from the World Health Organization (WHO 2010), the World Bank, and two UN agencies released a different set of figures. They calculated a slightly worse set of current figures for maternal mortality worldwide, but because they had started from a dramatically worse baseline, they also suggested a steeper rate of improvement over the previous two decades. In both the WHO and the IHME publications, the authors used an indicator called the maternal mortality ratio—that is, a ratio of maternal deaths to total live births—to report progress (fig. 2.1).[1]

Each set of estimates had its detractors. Prominent researchers criticized the *Lancet* paper for a rushed peer review process, a scramble intended to get the estimates out before the G8 meetings in which maternal health was to be a special focus. The *Lancet*'s editor criticized the critics, suggesting that they had advocated withholding good news for political reasons and pointing out that the WHO figures were not subjected to peer review at all (AbouZahr 2011). In the end which set of figures better reflects the reality of women's lives and deaths remains contested.

That controversy came to mind early in the dry season of 2013 as I talked with a longtime colleague, a member of the maternity teaching staff, at Queen Elizabeth Central Hospital. "Queens," as it is popularly known, is a large urban government hospital in Blantyre, Malawi. It is both a district hospital—meaning that people from the city attend it for anything that cannot be handled at the small nurse-run health centers stationed in the dense urban settlements nearby—and a referral hospital to which complex maternity cases from the southern third of the country may be sent. Many people are born at this hospital, if not as many as in its heyday: the estimate is approximately ten thousand a year now. Many people die, often prematurely. Births and deaths are all too frequently unattended when the woefully underresourced and understaffed nurse-midwives are attending to another patient—or to their paperwork, including the oversized blue ledgers where they are expected to record deaths in the maternity wing.[2] Years ago my colleague and I had worked together on the labor ward. In almost two years of biweekly maternal morbidity and mortality reviews back then, I never remember discussing morbidity: there was too much mortality to review.

Now we walked together up a sloping open-air corridor from a quiet block of offices toward the bustling wards, our shoes slipping a little on concrete floors polished by many, many feet. "They are saying that maternal mortality has dropped a lot, even to something like three hundred," my colleague said. "Wow," I responded. I too had heard some of this talk and was unsure whether to believe it; if true, it would be an extraordinary improvement. We stopped. Down the walkway toward us came a small procession. Two orderlies in white uniforms pushed a gurney on which a body lay shrouded in bright cloth. Behind them a middle-aged woman keened a sorrowful tune. I didn't catch all of the Chichewa, but I could hear "My sister, my sister." Behind her a small cluster of mourners sang in harmony, responses to her call. We stood still, heads slightly bowed. My colleague shook her head and spoke in a low voice: "They are saying we will meet the Millennium Development Goal. But I can't believe it. If it's that low, why are we still seeing this kind of thing every day?" The sad procession had passed now, and my colleague continued. "I think it has to be at least in the five hundred or six hundred range still. You know, there's a lot of pressure on this goal. A lot. The president has really staked her legitimacy on improving maternal mortality."

Why Do Numbers Matter?

One conversation happened in the hallway of an urban African hospital. The other took place in the pages of a prominent medical journal, published in the metropole of what was once the British Empire and distributed through the postcolonial world of which Queens Hospital is one small part. Both conversations feature numbers as points of anxiety and controversy. Together they suggest the importance and the complexities of metrics in what we now call global health. In this chapter I discuss why numbers matter and the difficulty with evidence (drawing on research in Malawi). I offer a close reading of the equations used in places like Malawi and in journals like the *Lancet* to produce these numbers, and an exploration of the epistemologies that inform those equations.

Health threats are powerful prods to political action because health is one of those rare goals that is broadly shared even by people who disagree on most other matters. Walls and borders do not keep out contaminated air or water quite as effectively as they keep out people. Infectious diseases and antibiotic-resistant superbugs get swapped readily in the places where we eat and work and especially in the places where we seek treatment for our ills. In other words, many health threats cannot be effectively contained to one marginalized—and thus readily disregarded—part of the human community. The richest can keep many threats at bay, but few people are wealthy enough to segregate themselves so thoroughly or to purchase their way to health. We humans share vulnerability to sickness and suffering, although the distribution of these experiences is starkly unequal; we also share the inevitability of death, although when we may most likely expect it is also unequal. Appeals to protect, promote, and preserve the public's health can be politically potent, then, drawing together broad coalitions. Indeed the protection of health has become one of the only politically justifiable checks on profit extraction in the era of late capitalism.

Health issues become political issues, and sometimes become actual policy, in at least two ways. We might think of the post hoc preventative regulations put in place after a disaster of some sort. In the United States readers might consider occupational safety measures after the Triangle Shirtwaist Factory fire; Europeans will recall the new rules for cattle feeding, transport, and slaughter imposed after a wave of human deaths from bovine spongiform encephalopathy ("mad cow disease"). But health policy is also prompted by health indicators: epidemiologists' calculations of births, deaths, and quality and quantity of life for a given population. These figures are sources of national pride and embarrassment, prompts for target setting, goads to new legislation and resource reallocation (see Oni-Orisan, this volume). A CNN story, "Doubling of Maternal Deaths in U.S. 'Scandalous,' Rights Group Says," cites an Amnesty International representative urging President Obama to act on these terrible numbers and a prominent academic obstetrician calling the figures "a national disgrace and a call to action" (Smith 2010). Such headlines appear in Malawi too, where they are used regularly to chastise — and sometimes to praise — political leaders.

Where disasters can prompt policy change through their emotional impact, health indicators work in part through an appearance of impartial objectivity. Crump (1990: 148) argued that numerical institutions (such as place-value notation) diffuse readily and are incorporated quickly into disparate contexts because they make "few demands on any local culture": they translate readily and appear transparently useful across realms. Health indicators serve similarly as a common numerical language among a wide range of experts, advocates, and bureaucrats working in the arena of health policy. Calculated as rates, ratios, and percentages, health indicators quantify the qualitative experience of human life: they convert people into abstractions, which is at once their major function, their strength, and their most troubling characteristic. They make order — but not just any order — from chaos. As Adams (2005) has noted, following Hacking (1990) and others, numbers are read as apolitical and morally neutral, which is precisely why they can be mobilized so effectively for moral and political projects. Numbers like mortality ratios and fertility rates get read as facts that can advance some political agendas and subvert others, facts that can alter people's perceptions of their own and others' lives (Kaufert and O'Neil 1990).

Health indicators suit the technical managerial logic of contemporary global public health because they can be tracked, graphed, compared across time and space, and statistically manipulated in ways that people cannot. These numbers speak of health in the language of business. They can be converted to dollars, inserted into equations that triage the alleviation of suffering and the postponement of death based on cost; this is the entire function of a whole category of indicators called health-adjusted life years, in which various kinds of sickness are converted to fractions of life or death, as are "unproductive" parts of life like old age and childhood. Health indicators have many uses. Most of those uses rest upon their claim to represent (in aggregate) actual people.[3] How they work, what they reveal, and what they conceal matters.

Maternal mortality numbers, the ratios estimated by the WHO and the IHME and spoken of in the halls at Queens, matter too. Just how bad is maternal mortality? Is it rising or falling? How fast? These numbers matter most obviously because they claim to represent deaths of actual people and because each death of a pregnant, laboring, or postpartum woman robs the world of a unique individual and leaves kin and friends to grieve. But the maternal mortality ratio matters to policymakers and health planners for at least three other reasons too.

First, the long stagnation in this most critical measure of maternal health has been understood by many observers as an indictment of gender inequity and of inequities between rich and poor. The gap between maternal mortality in wealthy nations and that in poor nations is greater than it is for any other health indicator. The magnitude and persistence of that gap are often read as symptoms of a widespread disregard for poor women's lives; that diagnosis is why the lack of progress toward meeting Millennium Development Goal 5 could be seen as a disfiguring scar on an imagined global body.

Second, in Malawi and many places nearby, dramatic disruptions of reproduction—such as excess stillbirths and abortions, drought and failed harvests, widespread infertility—have long been understood to be indicators of political illegitimacy (Kaspin 1996; Schoffeleers 2000). Good harvests and smooth reproduction indicate righteous leadership, and maternal death can therefore have serious political implications.

Third, maternal mortality is widely considered a sensitive indicator of a health system's overall functioning. Life-threatening obstetric emergencies happen at any time of the day or night, in any weather or season, often in extremely inconvenient places. They have multiple causes. They require knowledgeable and capable clinicians to understand what is happening and to respond quickly with a range of interventions (including transfusion, surgery, administration of magnesium sulfate, vacuum extraction, etc.) to stave off death. Therefore they require a level of basic effective health care infrastructure and personnel that is not as essential to certain other indicators, such as vaccination rates. Vertical and magic-bullet interventions are very unlikely to have much impact.

These numbers are important, then. Numbers like maternal mortality ratio estimates flatten messy events, render narratives legible, make unlike situations comparable. For that reason they are taken up readily in many domains, used by many parties for many purposes (Bowker and Star 1999; Porter 1992).[4] Most of the story that follows is about how numbers are made into legitimate evidence. The trouble with health indicators like the maternal mortality ratio, I will argue, involves problems of evidence, of epistemology, and of effect.

Evidence First

Accurate health indicators require a robust infrastructure of surveillance and audit. There is a teleology here: problems can be seen and tracked only if they are already understood to be important. As Julie Livingston (2012) has noted, for instance, because cancer in Africa was for so long thought not to be a problem, the surveillance necessary to determine that it was a problem was never developed. Measurement infrastructures tend to be particularly weak where threats to health and life are particularly severe (Mathers and Boerma 2010) — especially places where the fragmentation or total dissolution of medical care and governance produce what Peter Redfield (2006: 12) calls "the statistical vacuum of political collapse."

A case study can make clearer the problems with evidence and measurement and how those are exacerbated by an attenuated health system. So let us return to Queens Hospital, this time to a day a few years earlier than the hallway conversation described above, when a fifteen-year-old Malawian girl died. She had been transferred to Queens from a place I will call Kamudzi Health Center.[5] Like Malawi's hundreds of other health centers, Kamudzi combines outpatient clinics with a maternity ward. About a quarter of births in Malawi happen in health center maternity units.[6] With no surgical and very limited medical capacity, these units are intended to be the first line for antenatal care, low-acuity outpatient visits, normal births, and routine infant and child health care. The girl's "health passport," a small booklet in which her medical records were written, indicated that she had visited the health center twice during her pregnancy. One visit involved a single dose of medications for malaria. This was a presumptive diagnosis based on her report of fever and general body pains; her temperature was not taken and no malaria testing was done. The other was a routine prenatal visit. Her weight was recorded as normal; growth of the fetus as measured by the midwife's hands was also normal. Complications of hypertension are common in pregnancy, especially in teenagers, but her blood pressure was not recorded at either visit.

The girl came back to the health center in labor and had a normal delivery of a live infant. Immediately afterward she began to seize. Kamudzi Health Center, like most health centers, had no drugs to stop seizures. It had no diagnostic equipment except that necessary to spin a hematocrit and to get an HIV test. It had no working thermometer or blood pressure cuff. In other words, there was no way to conduct basic investigations of what might be going wrong and very little with which to intervene, even empirically. The nurse called for help, but there was only one working ambulance for this city of over 1.5 million people. During the two hours it took to arrive, the young mother had five seizures. She was comatose when she was bundled into the ambulance, and dead when she was taken out of it at Queens.

How might one explain this death? The nurse at the health center suspected eclampsia, a complication of high blood pressure that can cause swelling of the brain and seizures. At the maternal mortality review I attended, one of the interns pointed out that cerebral malaria can also cause seizures. That alternative diagnosis matters because epidemiologists would not count a cerebral malaria death as a maternal death; it has nothing to do with the pregnancy or its management.[7] One of our obstetricians had another explanation for deaths that occurred among very young women. "We didn't see this much in the old days," he said. "Some people believe this is a new problem with the advent of so-called democracy." In the pre-democracy past, claimed this man and several of the other older adults who spoke with me, the social control exerted by elders meant a fifteen-year-old girl would never have become pregnant in the first place.[8]

I do not know whether the girl had also consulted a local birth attendant, an herbalist in her village, or a church elder about her pregnancy, although such consultations are more the norm than not. In Malawi demographers estimate that somewhere around a quarter to a third of births occur at home or at the compound of an *mzamba* (Ministry of Health, Republic of Malawi 2010; National Statistical Office and ICF Macro 2011). *Azamba* (the plural or honorific form) are people who are called on in their commu-

nities to attend births, some of whom have a great deal of practical experience and some of whom have almost none, some of whom have a little biomedical training and some of whom have none.[9] Antenatal consultations
with *azamba*, herbalists, and other healers are even more common than are
births entrusted to them.

Having talked to quite a few *azamba* and herbalists, I know they would
likely advance another explanation for her death: the path for birth was
not ready. The girl's body was not yet mature enough to handle pregnancy, much as a field is not ready for a crop until it has been cultivated
and cleared of weeds. Some obstetricians would agree; the profession has a
long history of trying to predict who is and is not suited to deliver by using
pelvic X-rays, especially in adolescents. Other professions share some of
this concern. Many biological anthropologists, for instance, consider complicated delivery to be an unfortunate consequence of human evolution:
the reshaping of the pelvis resulting from bipedal locomotion, in combination with the brain growth that produces big fetal heads.

Which narrative is most plausible, which story most usable, and to what
end? Was her death from malaria? Cerebral edema? An unready path? Bi-
pedalism? The national poverty that meant there was no blood pressure
cuff at the clinic and not enough ambulances to move her quickly to the
hospital? Teen pregnancy? Democracy? How far back do we look in time?
On what scale do we think: the individual, the social, the national, the
species? How might the team reviewing this case record her death, how
might that death figure into health statistics, and how will those indicators
then be used to prescribe (or proscribe) certain kinds of interventions?

Body Counts and Death Estimates

Ideally one would calculate maternal mortality by counting every maternal
death and every live birth in a given population to produce a simple ratio
called the maternal mortality ratio, or MMR:[10]

MMR = maternal deaths / live births x 100,000

The world's lowest national-level MMRs are in the single digits. The
global average is thought to be in the mid-200s. When my colleague estimated Malawi's maternal mortality at 500 or 600, the MMR is the number
to which she was referring. But there is no effective vital registration sys-

tem in Malawi. Families and villages may report a birth or a death but were not required to do so by law until quite recently (2009); many remain unaware of the obligation, and of those who are aware, few can pay the fee for a death certificate, equivalent to about forty days of work at minimum wage. Clinics and hospitals are expected to report gross numbers of births and deaths, but it is not so easy to keep track of the numbers, and they often go astray. Efforts to track maternal death cases have had mixed results. It is often estimated that more than three quarters of deaths in Malawi are never recorded anywhere (e.g., Singogo et al. 2013). The fifteen-year-old's death turns out to be one of them; the case records that the department had painstakingly compiled during our biweekly reviews never made it to the Ministry of Health, and I found out later that our district reported no maternal deaths at all for the year.

So in the absence of reliable data, the "measurement" of maternal mortality in places like Malawi is really an estimate of mortality. The most common way to estimate—common because it is inexpensive—draws from a demographic and health survey that takes place every five to ten years in many poor countries.[11] For those countries that include a "sisterhood module" in their surveys, research assistants ask a sample of people to recall the lives and deaths of each sibling. If a dead sibling was a sister and at least twelve years old when she died, the interviewer asks whether she had been pregnant at the time or within two months of death.[12] The survey respondents' responses, as recorded by field surveyors, are then weighted and extrapolated by statisticians to represent the nation. Data from sisterhood surveys account for over 80 percent of the maternal mortality estimates that the WHO used in sub-Saharan Africa; globally sisterhood surveys run a distant second to vital registration systems in providing estimates of maternal deaths. As the last step in the estimating process, demographers and epidemiologists work with computerized statistical models to input what data are available (sisterhood surveys, targeted surveillance reports, surveys of recent deaths, etc.), adjust those data in an attempt to compensate for suspected under- or overreporting, throw out data deemed too far off to be plausible, impute data where none are available, and estimate uncertainty ranges of both deaths that are counted and death rates that are imputed.

The model used to estimate maternal mortality by the WHO consortium will give you a sense of how these equations work:

$$\log(PM_i^{na}) = \beta_0 + \beta_1\log(GDP_i) + \beta_2\log(GFR_i) + \beta_3SAB_i + \alpha^c_{j[i]} + \alpha^R_{k[i]} + \varepsilon_i$$

PM_i^{na} = proportion of maternal deaths among non-AIDS deaths in women 15–49

GDP_i = gross domestic product per capita (2005 PPP dollars[13])

GFR_i = general fertility rate (live births per woman aged 15–49)

SAB_i = skilled attendant at birth (proportion of all births)

$\alpha^c_{j[i]}$ = variable intercept component for country j

$\alpha^R_{k[i]}$ = variable intercept component for region k

ε_i = error

This regression equation may at first appear daunting. But even before attending to the mathematics of it, there are some interesting things to look at—and looking reveals where problems of evidence begin to shade into problems of epistemology.

First, note that every number put into this equation in Malawi and places like it is an estimate, not a count. This equation draws on six estimated numbers (everything after the equals sign but the "error" figure ε_i) to smooth estimates derived from sisterhood surveys.[14] The sisterhood survey estimates (already weighted to match the presumed demographics of the nation as a whole) are first increased by 10 percent, a proportion thought to compensate for the underreporting that happens due to secrecy or obliviousness about abortion-related and other early pregnancy deaths. They are then decreased by a specified percentage, a proportion intended to account for deaths that happened during pregnancy but are not really "maternal," such as cerebral malaria deaths. The decrease is 10 percent in sub-Saharan Africa, 15 percent in all other parts of the world.[15] The formula produces an estimate of the proportion of deaths among HIV-negative women of reproductive age (assumed to be between fifteen and forty-nine years) that are maternal deaths. Maternal death is more effectively estimated as a proportion than as a number, because deaths of reproductive-age women are generally underreported in sibling histories and sisterhood surveys, while live births are not. A calculation of MMR based on underreported pregnancy-related deaths / correctly reported births x 100,000 will result in an incorrectly low estimate of maternal death. However, studies also suggest that the degree of underreporting is similar for pregnancy-related deaths and deaths not related to pregnancy among women ages fifteen to forty-nine. Therefore a *proportion* of deaths in this age group during or just after pregnancy, underreported pregnancy-related deaths / underreported total deaths, will be less distorted and can in theory be combined with population figures to get a more accurate picture of maternal mortality. To get from this proportion to an MMR involves four additional estimates. First, estimated AIDS-related maternal deaths are added in to produce PM, the proportion of deaths considered "maternal" among all deaths in women age fifteen to forty-nine.[16] Finally:

$$PM \, (D/B) \times 100,000 = MMR$$

D = number of deaths overall in women ages 15–49, calculated from WHO estimated death rates and UN Development Program (UNDP) population estimates

B = number of live births, an estimate taken from other UNDP databases

Each estimate has its own sources of uncertainty and bias, making the final product—an MMR number that looks like and gets used as a solid fact—quite a wobbly figure indeed. Even the estimates of uncertainty ranges around the figures entail their own uncertainties, as those closest to the calculations will most readily admit. In fact as the UN-WHO team that developed the model reports, three of the four numbers used to calculate paradoxically precise-looking uncertainty intervals were "based mostly on our own intuition, as appropriate empirical evidence is lacking" (Wilmoth et al. 2012: 23).

So the first thing to note is that every number put into this equation is an estimate, and several are products of multiple estimates. Second, consider which estimated numbers get included as contributing factors (boldface) and which possible contributors do not:

$$\log(PM_i^{na}) = \beta_0 + \beta_1 \log(\textbf{GDP}_i) + \beta_2 \log(\textbf{GFR}_i) + \beta_3 \textbf{SAB}_i + \alpha^c_{j[i]} + \alpha^R_{k[i]} + \varepsilon_i$$

The WHO's equation uses three covariates, also called explanatory variables, to estimate maternal mortality. The two weighted most heavily are per capita gross domestic product and general fertility rate. Each of these is known to have a substantial correlation with maternal mortality in data from countries where births and deaths are actually counted. The third is "skilled attendance at birth," which actually refers not to skill but to apparent job classification. All attendants believed by delivering women to be doctors or nurses are counted as skilled; all others are counted as unskilled. One of the most interesting things about this variable is that it has never been conclusively demonstrated to the satisfaction of epidemiologists that skilled attendance at birth matters to maternal mortality, although nearly everyone—policymakers, village women, doctors—assumes that it does and although the historical evidence for its importance is quite compelling. It is possible that the presence of skilled attendants matters little where health care infrastructure is badly broken down and crucial resources rarely available, as in the death of the fifteen-year-old. (I will return to this question later.) In fact the IHME model did not include skilled birth attendance as an explanatory variable, although researchers there speculated that some of the covariates they did include (such as newborn deaths) were proxies for skilled attendance at birth.

Modeled Numbers: Irrelevant, Powerful, or Tautological?

In sixty-one of the sixty-five countries where vital registration systems are more or less complete, this model is not used at all. Instead reported deaths are simply adjusted for suspected underreporting—typically by multiplying all numbers by 1.5—and the resulting lines are "smoothed," as the graph for the United States in figure 2.2 shows.

The model *is* used for four countries with good vital registration systems in which a combination of small population and rare maternal deaths (or, as the WHO sometimes refers to them, "maternal mortality events") makes trends look erratic. In Iceland, for instance, with only four thousand or five thousand births a year, in the absence of such data smoothing maternal mortality ratios appear to jump dramatically every year that one maternal death is reported, remaining at zero in the majority of years when no deaths are reported.[17]

The model becomes more important in the eighty-eight countries—including Malawi—that do not have functional vital registration systems but do have one or more estimates of maternal mortality from surveys using sisterhood methods or other sources. In these the model is used to fill in data that don't exist, smooth out data that do, and throw out data that are such a poor fit that they are deemed unlikely to be true. You can see the process at work in figure 2.3. The points indicate actual estimates from demographic and health surveys; the solid line indicates the modeled estimates that got published as Malawi's maternal mortality; dashed lines indicate the uncertainty range. If one simply accepted the sisterhood numbers at face value here, maternal mortality would show an overall small rise

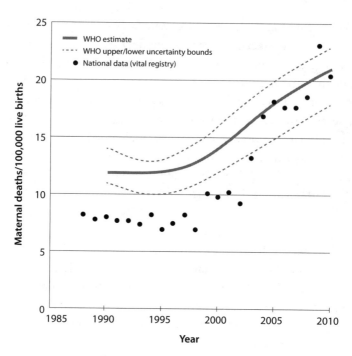

FIGURE 2.2 · WHO maternal mortality estimates for the United States, 1990–2010.

Sources: WHO, UNICEF, UNFPPA, World Bank, UN Population Division Maternal Mortality Estimation Inter-agency Group, "Maternal Mortality in 1990–2010: United States of America," http://www.who.int/gho/maternal_health/countries/usa.xls (where the original chart may be seen) and the U.S. National Vital Statistics System.

between 1990 and 2010, with a particular exacerbation in the late 1990s and early 2000s. But the modeled estimate tells a different story, of steady if slow progress that has become more rapid since 1996 or so.

The model becomes a tautology in the twenty-seven countries for which no data exist at all; for instance, WHO figures show an impressive decline in maternal mortality in Equatorial Guinea, which has had no national measure or count of maternal deaths for over twenty years, because the GDP rose with rising oil prices and GDP is such an important variable in the equation (see figure 2.4).[18]

What is the point of this equation? As demographers and statisticians develop a model like this, they are looking for the single equation that best explains all the variability seen in measures of maternal mortality. Such an equation is pleasing in its parsimony. Beyond its aesthetic pleasures, it has practical uses: it allows more confident predictions of likely health indica-

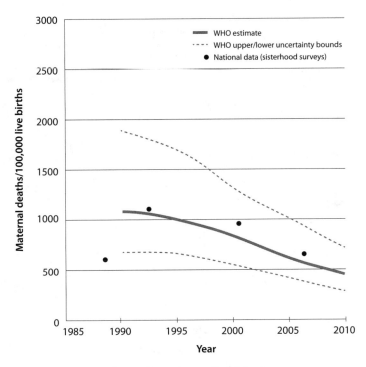

FIGURE 2.3 · WHO maternal mortality estimates for Malawi, 1990–2010.

Source: WHO, UNICEF, UNFPPA, World Bank, UN Population Division Maternal Mortality
Estimation Inter-agency Group, "Maternal Mortality in 1990–2010: Malawi," http://www.who
.int/gho/maternal_health/countries/mwi.xls (where the original chart may be seen).

tors where health indicators are lacking, which can then be used to coax
resources from governments and funders. It can also lead epidemiologists
to be suspicious of certain estimates or counts of maternal mortality that
are far from what the model predicts — even if these counts would be politically useful to certain interested parties. If correlations with certain covariates (such as GDP or SAB) are strong, it can suggest plausible interventions
for better maternal survival.

Given the importance of the model, we might note some variables
that are not in the equation: any indicator of political stability (although
it appears that chronic civil and international conflict are huge drivers of
mortality in places like Afghanistan and the Democratic Republic of the
Congo); any indicator of income or gender inequality; any indicator of
state funding for health care. Most striking to me is the absence of anything
that might measure the quality of care once women are inside the build-

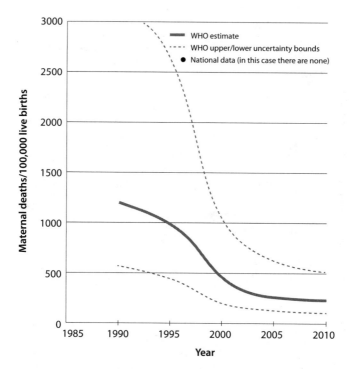

FIGURE 2.4 · WHO maternal mortality estimates for Equatorial Guinea, 1990–2010.

Source: WHO, UNICEF, UNFPPA, World Bank, UN Population Division Maternal Mortality
Estimation Inter-agency Group, "Maternal Mortality in 1990–2010: Equatorial Guinea," http://
www.who.int/gho/maternal_health/countries/gnq.xls (where the original chart may be seen).

ings marked as medical spaces and in the hands of those people marked as
skilled attendants.

Other interesting assumptions are also at work here. The process of regression in general and the logarithmic transformation made in this particular equation are largely about smoothing.[19] The idea is that the best
line through all these points is a smooth line that is nonetheless not too far
away from any point not disregarded as an implausible outlier. Why should
that be true? Might we not expect a less smooth line for, say, Sierra Leone,
in which a vicious civil war finally ended in 2002, or Rwanda, in which a
huge chunk of the population was slaughtered in 1994? If visibly pregnant
women were particular targets of violence, or even if their access to decent
health care was especially constrained during such conflicts, is it not plausible to expect abrupt changes in maternal deaths? The beta-coefficients,
estimates of the magnitude by which GDP, GFR, and SAB change maternal

real
life isn't
smooth

72 · Claire L. Wendland

mortality, are the same for every country in the world, while "region" (in this case the UN administrative region used to track changes relevant to the Millennium Development Goals) and "country" are black-box constants, kept separate from the variables.[20] One can imagine other ways of modeling that might have different results and different implications: What if skilled attendance at birth matters less in regions where skilled attendants are usually working without adequate health care infrastructure (ambulances, drugs, blood banks), as we might expect? What if fertility matters more in regions with extremely high surgical delivery rates (as we might expect, given that mortality rises with repeat cesarean sections)? These critical questions are hidden by the practices of calculation embedded in mortality estimation models. Crump (1990: 148–49), who described how quickly certain ways of using numbers spread, also noted that they can be Trojan horses. While numerical practices function readily across very different cultural contexts, he argued, their support for particular kinds of institutions eventually makes those institutions dominant. In this case the statistical infrastructure of mortality modeling makes certain ways of *thinking* dominant by embedding them in the architecture of epidemiology.

Other features of health indicators as a category are epistemologically curious. One: most require denominators (percentage of whom? ratio of what?), and those denominators designate the most important relations among people as territorial ones. Geographically bounded, institutionally legible spaces, like zip codes or nations, substitute for communities. We can see that in the regression equation: two of the numbers used to model maternal mortality are additions to the Y-intercept specific to the country and the region. Two: the uncounted don't count. Many health indicators exclude prison inmates, for instance, meaning that such measures as HIV rates can look very different in indicators than they do in people's social networks or in local hospitals. Three: health itself gets conceptualized as a standard monolith from which chunks can be chipped away by premature death—or by other kinds of specified suffering that are converted into globally standardized fractions of death called quality-adjusted life years and disability-adjusted life years (Gold et al. 2002). And four: even when health is defined capaciously as human flourishing, experiences that profoundly affect human flourishing—the loss of a child, imprisonment, the inability to secure housing or employment, bearing witness to repeated trauma—get relegated to development (and not health) indicators, if they are indicators at all.

In addition to what they leave out and what they presume, metrics have other effects about which we might be concerned. All too often the indicators themselves become the focus of attention. In India, as Veena Das (1999) notes, the attention to vaccination rates meant that no one was accountable for considering adverse vaccine reactions or for adverse consequences of strategies to boost rates, such as withholding birth certificates and therefore all social services from unvaccinated infants. "Skilled attendance at birth" has been the most important indicator of maternal health care functioning (or "process indicator," in public health terminology) for a long time. The focus on skilled birth attendance has led to outlawing of other kinds of birth attendants in many locations, not always with positive consequences. It has also led to an emphasis on the people needed for institutionalized birth and a considerably lower priority placed on the tools and infrastructure those people need to deploy (or even maintain) their skills. When indicators themselves are fetishes, the root causes of the problems they are meant to document fade from view and options for addressing them are prematurely foreclosed (Porter 1995). And here we can finally get back to my colleague's worry that the president's legitimacy was staked on Malawi's maternal mortality ratio.

Joyce Banda assumed the presidency of Malawi in 2012, during a time of great upheaval after the incumbent suddenly died. Unelected—and a woman to boot—she promptly made several extremely unpopular decisions intended to restore the flow of foreign aid to Malawi and resulting in the short term in considerable suffering for many Malawians. Her signature domestic policy initiatives centered on women's health; in particular she made strong efforts to tackle Malawi's maternal mortality problem. She corralled donor funds to build maternity waiting homes in which women with pregnancies designated as high risk can wait for labor nearer to a hospital. She authorized—indeed ordered—chiefs to improve maternal health in their districts. (While chiefs have employed a number of strategies, including several quite creative approaches, some of these efforts have involved punishing fines for anyone reporting a maternal death.) And she reaped repeated acclaim for these efforts. We can see the focus on indicators in recent articles from one of Malawi's national newspapers.

In an article with the headline "Malawi Maternal Mortality Rate Reduced—Chief Kwataine," Thokozani Mbewe reported in April 2013 as follows:

Presidential Initiative on Safe Motherhood and Maternal Health chairperson Senior Chief Kwataine has painted a rosy picture on reducing the country's maternal mortality rate.

Chief Kwataine reported that since the launch of the Presidential Initiative on Safe motherhood and maternal health last year by President Joyce Banda, there has been a reduction in the maternal mortality from 675 out of 100,00 to 460 out of 100,00 women dying during childbirth.

As the deadline for reaching the Millennium Development Goals approaches, Kwataine is confident that Malawi will meet its target by 2015.[21]

Accompanying the article, a full-color photo showed Banda, in an outfit featuring the orange color associated with her political party, speaking with several male chiefs. Two months later a press release from the Malawi News Agency reported external approval for Banda on a diplomatic visit to Japan:

Malawi President Joyce Banda on Saturday received a loud applause and standing ovation on her approach of involving traditional leaders in the fight against maternal mortality through her Presidential [initiative] on safe motherhood in Malawi.

This has resulted in the dropping of maternal deaths from 675 to 460 per every 100 000 live births.

"Your Excellencies, distinguished ladies and gentlemen, my strategy has received significant support from all stakeholders and is showing encouraging results," stressed Banda during her key note address at a symposium.[22]

One thing these articles show is how numbers act as fetishes, inanimate things imbued with power. The number-as-fetish is particularly evident in the first excerpt, which cites MMR figures as painting "a rosy picture" of improved maternal health without any clarity on what they actually are: the denominator given for the ratio is incorrect by a factor of ten, and seems to refer to numbers of women giving birth rather than numbers of live births. It is also evident—if less blatantly so—in the second article, which cites the numbers accurately but without crucial context. While Banda's efforts to improve maternal mortality were important, overdue, and interesting, they could not in any way be related to the apparent decline in maternal mortality that the president's spokespersons cited. That decline, which was

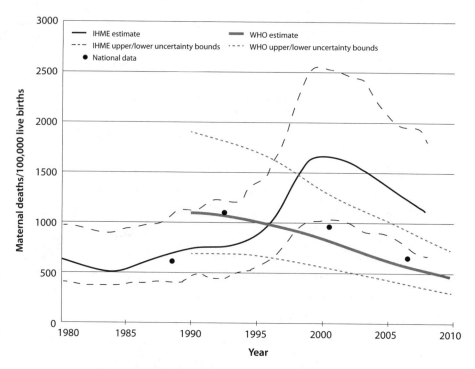

FIGURE 2.5 · Two statistical stories about maternal death trends in Malawi.

Sources: Hogan et al. 2010, online data supplement 171; World Health Organization 2010.

calculated based on surveys collected in 2010, two years before she took power, uses an estimating method that relies on data from the seven-year range before that (National Statistical Office and ICF Macro 2011).

The timing is not the only problem. Both articles cite the same numbers: the president's initiative "resulted in the dropping of maternal deaths from 675 to 460 per 100 000 live births." A review of the UN-WHO graph for Malawi (fig. 2.3) shows the source of both numbers. The 675 is derived from survey data obtained in 2010 and covering the seven years prior. (It seems to have been located on the x axis at 2006.5, the midpoint of this range.) The 460 is the modelers' extrapolation for 2010 from the regression equation "smoothing" that same data point. These are apples and oranges, not comparable numbers.

Finally, the indicators the newspapers cite are not the only versions out there. Figure 2.5 shows how the IHME transformed the same basic data into a very different account of what was happening to maternal death in Malawi.

The Power of a Numerical Story

Those closest to the production of health indicators like the maternal mortality ratio often recognize best the extent to which they are fictions, painstakingly crafted for verisimilitude but with an always uncertain relationship to verity. The team that developed the equation to which we have been attending described it in a methodology paper in terms more reminiscent of science fiction than of scientific statistics as nonstatisticians usually think about them. The authors concluded that it is "important to be modest and honest about the limitations of our knowledge. . . . *All existing estimates of levels and trends in maternal mortality provide no more than an image of a reality that may have been*" (Wilmoth et al. 2012: 33, my italics). Indicators have power in part because they make statistically—and politically—malleable stories in ways that individuals' lives do not (Erikson 2012; see also Oni-Orisan, this volume); lives and even clinical case reports usually reveal uncertainties that indicators *as they are actually used*, if not as they are described by their makers, conceal (Hodžić 2013).

Like an X-ray of a woman's pelvis, the equations that model maternal death render certain aspects of life and labor invisible and make others, normally hidden to ordinary nonexpert eyes, visible. Like X-rays and stories, equations may help us to see certain things we previously didn't see clearly, and like X-rays and stories, they do so by rendering other things transparent—that is, by making it possible for a viewer to see straight through those things and soon to forget them altogether.

But aspects of a life, a body, the experiences of a community are seen and seeable for many reasons. We can see—and carefully measure—bones on a pelvic X-ray not because bones are the most important thing that predicts whether an about-to-be-newborn's head gets stuck in its mother's pelvis or slides through easily but simply because bones are what the electromagnetic waves we call X-rays allow us to see. (The calcium atoms in bones absorb X-ray photons. The smaller atoms of soft tissues do not.) A statistical modeling equation for maternal mortality privileges method in similar ways. It allows epidemiologists to see some things because they can be measured and counted, at least in theory. Things that are not—or cannot be—made into numbers do not appear in equations, no matter how much they matter for a woman's chances of life or death, health or misery. These computerized narratives give heavier weights to some possible factors than others. They put these factors in relation to each other to predict an outcome ahead of time or to explain it after the fact.

The product of an equation looks like a number and works like a fact, but it is more like the moral of a story. In this case it is a story that bolsters the shaky foundations of a presidency. It is a story that hides uncertainty under layers of numbers, even when those numbers are estimates based on approximations based on intuitions, and even when those closest to the production of the numbers emphasize most their provisional nature. Equations are explanations that highlight some plot twists and ignore others, that emphasize certain actors and relegate others to the supporting cast, like any good story does.

These equations are powerful, and they are useful. Unlike most clinical case narratives, they can bring into the heart of medicine a way to consider just how powerfully economic and social forces affect people's bodies and just how often economic and social deprivation end people's lives. Health indicators like the maternal mortality ratio originated as ways to work toward progress, to track and reform the ills of social life. George Canguilhem (1991: 161) famously claimed that each society has "the mortality that suits it," that statistical profiles of death give evidence of political decisions about equality and justice, about whose lives count and whose do not. We might think too of the *Lancet* editorialist who called limited progress on maternal mortality a deforming scar on the body of global health, thus reembodying a disembodied set of numbers. I do not wish to claim that politicizing maternal mortality ratios is a bad thing to do. In a world in which good governance is measured in numbers, it is probably the single most important way to begin improving maternal health. But if maternal mortality numbers and their production hide (rather than foreground) deficits of health care infrastructure and its funding and maintenance, then the particular kinds of political work they prompt are likely to be less effective than they might be. Rather than working to improve the skills of the less skilled, and providing the already skilled with the tools they need to do their work well, one makes a presidential legacy out of empowering already powerful chiefs and disempowering already marginalized *azamba*.

The equations that model maternal mortality in Malawi and places like it are important, however provisional and uncertain they are. But their provisionality and uncertainty is part of what is important about them. This chapter is not intended to provoke disdain for such attempts at estimating death. I intend simply to show how they act, like the nurses' stories, the doctors' radiographs, and the explanations of herbalists and *azamba*, to reveal some things clearly and to hide others—and how these stories, like others, become active in the world. It is when we fail to recognize them as partial, created, fallible stories that the metrics of global health are especially troubling.

Notes

1. I will refer to the groups as the IHME and the WHO for clarity and brevity, but the latter was really a multiagency team called the United Nations Maternal Mortality Estimation Inter-agency Group. Their findings were published by the WHO.

2. Nearly all births, including complex ones involving twins, breech deliveries, and vacuum extractions, are the responsibility of nurse-midwives and students. Obstetricians, generalist doctors, and the surgically trained midlevel clinicians known in Malawi as "clinical officers" typically attend only surgical deliveries, although they are (at least in theory) available to consult on complex obstetric cases.

3. But not all of them. Erikson (2012) notes that health indicators also serve as a new kind of commodity, one that helps money move, makes the chaotic appear manageable and the dysfunctional functional, and allows one to "improve global health" for populations at a spatial and temporal remove from actual (infectious, distressing, needy, or inexplicable) people.

4. Thanks to Linda Hogle for reminding me how important this part of the story is, even though this short chapter does not do it justice. See Adams (2005) for a fascinating example of what happens when maternal mortality ratios serve as the primary (and perhaps the only) common intellectual currency among funders, researchers, and officials.

5. Kamudzi is a pseudonym. I am not able to use a pseudonym for Queens.

6. The most recent Ministry of Health (2010) estimates indicate that 25 percent of births happen in health centers, 40 percent in hospitals, and 35 percent outside of health facilities (whether at home or elsewhere).

7. Eclampsia and cerebral malaria are by no means the only diagnostic possibilities in a biomedical framework, although from a medical perspective they are probably the likeliest in a Malawian teenager. A review article on neurological emergencies in pregnancy mentions at least eleven possible causes for seizure, most but not all of them exacerbated by pregnancy (Edlow et al. 2013). Presumably intended for first-world medical audiences, the article does not list malaria.

8. As Kaler (2001) has noted, however, older Malawian adults' reminiscences about a past understood to be more morally upright appear to be important ways of expressing discontent about the present. Kaler's work on the so-called decline of marriage shows little difference between discussions of that decline in the late 1990s and in archived material from the early twentieth century. It appears that conflicting moral claims get worked out in the language of sexuality, sexual infractions, and the problematic sexuality of young people.

9. In global health parlance these people are usually referred to as TBAs (traditional birth attendants). I use one of the local terms instead because it is not clear to me how

substantial the overlap is between those people called—by themselves or by women who use them—*azamba* and those characterized by Ministry of Health officials as TBAS. As other anthropologists have noted, the TBA can be an elusive category (Langwick 2012; Pigg 1997).

10. While epidemiologists refer to this ratio as addressing a population, in practice the calculations are done on a place: the numbers of births and deaths are counted (or estimated) for a bounded territory into and out of which people may be moving. Location stands in for population. Live births are not the perfect denominator here, as pregnancies that do not end in live births (e.g., ectopic pregnancies, stillbirths, abortions) also pose risks for pregnant women. They are the denominator easiest to obtain from vital registries, censuses, and household surveys, however.

11. In Malawi and seventy-four other countries these demographic and health surveys are based on modules developed by a large and profitable corporation, ICF Macro / ICF International, based in Washington DC. The company continues to provide technical assistance and analytical services. As Merry (2011) notes, indicators produced through these surveys are excellent examples of the blurring of private and public, academic and corporate, national and transnational that often characterizes technologies of contemporary governance.

12. Official definitions draw a boundary at forty-two days after the end of pregnancy for a death to count as "maternal." In practice two months has proven to be a more reasonable duration for field interviewers to ask about and their respondents to remember.

13. Purchasing power parity dollars: national currency converted to U.S. dollars and adjusted to indicate its ability to purchase a standard "basket" of goods and services, in recognition that a tomato may be much less expensive in Malawi while a car may be more expensive.

14. The presence of the error figure in the equation is a textual acknowledgment of the data's limitation. It is a reminder that the *true* value of the dependent variable PM_i^{na} is the product of the equation plus an unknown error. When the model is used with actual estimates of PM_i^{na} derived from field surveys, ε_i can be useful in estimating the bounds of uncertainty. For predictive purposes, however, ε_i is a sort of ghost figure, a haunting but ethereal reminder of the unknown; when the equation is actually used to *predict* PM_i^{na}, ε_i's value must be set to zero.

15. At the end of this increase-and-decrease procedure, for Malawi and other sub-Saharan African nations, the sisterhood numbers are pretty much where they started (Wilmoth et al. 2012).

16. I will not go into the details of this calculation here, but it may be worth noting that the WHO and IHME teams made completely different assumptions about how AIDS might be contributing to maternal death. (The IHME, for instance, assumed that pregnant and nonpregnant women were equally likely to die of AIDS. The WHO group assumed that pregnant women were 60 percent *less* likely to die of AIDS than nonpregnant women. The IHME counted all AIDS deaths in pregnant women as maternal; the WHO counted half of them.) The different approaches actually drew the two teams' final estimates closer together, although it made the trend lines each group provided for maternal deaths over time look more disparate. Interested readers are referred to

Wilmoth et al. (2012: 19–22, 31–33); the authors note honestly that the dearth of empirical data on AIDS and maternal death meant that they "were forced to choose values based on weak evidence in some cases and on no evidence at all in others" (20).

17. See WHO, UNICEF, UNFPPA, World Bank, UN Population Division Maternal Mortality Estimation Inter-agency Group, "Maternal Mortality in 1990–2010: Iceland," http://www.who.int/gho/maternal_health/countries/isl.xls for the WHO chart of maternal mortality in Iceland.

18. AbouZahr (2011) drew my attention to the case of Equatorial Guinea. It is dramatic, but it is not unique. The WHO lists Equatorial Guinea among the nations likely to meet Millennium Development Goal 5 based on this projection. United Nations documents feature it as the only nation in the world likely to meet Goal 5 but not Goal 4, which relates to child survival. Ironically the country is well known to demographers as an exemplary "poor health achiever," that is, a nation in which increased GDP has not translated into expected gains in health. Oil money has raised the GDP but has not improved life expectancy and infant survival (which rates, unlike maternal mortality, are estimated by the health ministry there) to match. One may reasonably expect that maternal mortality—which typically tracks roughly with neonatal mortality—has also lagged. Thanks to Monica Grant for alerting me to this point.

19. Using a logarithm allows one to treat variables that increase or decrease geometrically as if they were linear, which makes it easier to produce a smooth line.

20. β_0, which may look like a coefficient but is really a constant, is 2.253. β_1 is −0.217, β_2 is 1.272, and β_3 is −0.652. The negative numbers indicate that increases in skilled attendance at birth and in GDP are correlated with a decrease in maternal deaths, while the positive number indicates that rising fertility is correlated with more maternal deaths. For Malawi, the "region" constant α^R_k is 0.329 and the "country" constant α^c_j is −0.106 (Wilmoth et al. 2012, data supplement).

21. Thokozani Mbewe, "Malawi Maternal Mortality Reduced—Chief Kwataine," *Nyasa Times*, April 2, 2013, online.

22. Malawi News Agency, "Malawi Scores Highly on Maternal Health: JB Gets Standing Ovation in Japan," *Nyasa Times*, June 4, 2013, online.

3 · THE OBLIGATION TO COUNT The Politics of Monitoring
Maternal Mortality in Nigeria ADEOLA ONI-ORISAN

"The hospital is politically motivated," Dr. Oloke informed me amid the morning bustle of activity at the Hospital for Mothers and Children.[1] Women were lining up along the hospital's concrete walls, waiting for registration to open. Some carried babies tied to their backs with printed fabrics while others with rounded bellies shifted uncomfortably in place. Meanwhile the staff was setting up for what would be yet another day of tending to hundreds of women and children. Fresh-faced nurses in pastel-colored scrubs were taking over for their weary night-shift colleagues, and the doctors, including Dr. Oloke, were collecting in small groups according to rank, swapping stories about the previous night.

This morning there was troubling news to be shared. A woman had died overnight. Blessing, a forty-one-year-old mother of three, had delivered her fourth healthy baby at a police clinic nearby, but difficulty arose when it was time to deliver the placenta. The clinicians couldn't remove it entirely, so Blessing started to bleed uncontrollably, likely from where the torn placenta remained attached to her uterus. She was referred to the Hospital for Mothers and Children, but according to Dr. Oloke, she didn't arrive there until three hours later. When she finally arrived in a personal car, she was accompanied by her husband, some relatives, and a unit of blood meant to be transfused into her at the hospital. Dr. Oloke was waiting in the emergency room when Blessing was carried in. He recounted to me that just as he approached her he saw that she was "white, cold, gasped, and stopped breathing." He could do nothing more than declare her deceased.

Dr. Oloke had been called into the hospital chief medical director's office the next morning. "[Dr. Adetunde] read my documentation [and] concluded [Blessing] was dead even before she came in even though her last breath was in my presence," he told me as he walked out of the director's office. I asked him why the director would come to this conclusion, and it was then that he declared, "The hospital is politically motivated. . . . She would have been an *unnecessary* mortality."

It was the beginning of the month and the hospital was consequently preparing for its monthly mortality and morbidity review. This was a meeting that all the hospital employees, from doctors to gardeners, were expected to attend in order to review the hospital's performance and present the total number of mortalities for the previous month. These numbers would be used to tabulate the local government area's in-hospital maternal mortality rates. Since the hospital had only had one other death that month, adding Blessing's death would have doubled the maternal mortality rate. But because she had left the police clinic still breathing, she would not be added to their death toll. Thus her death wasn't counted. As far as the official health facility records and state government reports were concerned, Blessing didn't count.

The story of the death of Blessing is all too familiar. Similar anecdotes of maternal mortality are told in global health classrooms and conferences all over the world. Stories like these, with anonymized victims and struggling health care providers, have a way of emotionally priming listeners for the devastating numbers that will follow, the astounding rates at which women die giving birth in lower-income countries. Listeners are meant to multiply the story they have heard by the numbers of regional mortality rates that usually follow to arrive at the appropriate level of dismay, gaining a feeling of urgency in the process. The motivation to get involved among those who become aware of these statistics is often determined in relation to these emotion-laden calculations. Along the way from anecdotal cases to national statistics to global health textbooks, the sometimes staggering, sometimes subtle differences in the circumstances of each particular person who dies, each woman who does not make it through childbirth alive, are lost.

For example, formulations of causes of maternal death have been dramatically reduced to one or more of three delays. The "three-delays model," developed twenty years ago by Thaddeus and Maine (1994) and now widely accepted in the global maternal health world, is used as a tool to target interventions for preventing maternal mortality. According to Thaddeus and Maine, the three factors contributing to death after the onset of an obstetric complication are delay in the decision to seek care, delay in reaching appropriate care, and delay in receiving adequate care once in a health facility. The model has had a profound effect on practice, research, and the mobilization of funding. However, once applied generally to maternal mortality, this simplification to a set of temporal choices can obscure more complex understandings about the causes of maternal death and the routes to preventing them. The same can be said of maternal metrics.

Dr. Oloke's story is slightly more complete. His story and, in this case, that of Blessing suggest that the numbers do much more than account for death. They even do more than simply obscure the experiences of women in childbirth. His story tells us that as a result of the power that they are invested with, these numbers can become political instruments. Put another way, at times these numbers do a better job of reflecting a government's political goals than the facts of the situation they purport to tell us about.

In what follows I illustrate how the global health industry's dependence on specific kinds of quantitative knowledge—particularly numerical data in maternal health—structures and limits possibilities for both healing and local governance. I use ethnographic fieldwork on the recently established Healthy Mothers Healthy Babies (HMHB) program in a southwestern state in Nigeria to trace the impact of global public health agendas on local realities. My discussion is based on research interviews with doctors, nurses, patients, and government officials in HMHB health facilities, where I also engaged in ethnographic fieldwork.[2]

By exploring the close clinical encounters that are produced by the demand for clinicians to "see like a research project" (Biruk 2012) in the effort to comply with the demands of evidence-based global health, I highlight the ways health aid and the global health programs supported by it are far

from being either neutral or apolitical. I do not mean that global health programs are inherently political or that they use numbers to advance these
political goals (by now a commonplace insight in the political economy of
health literature). Rather I want to show how the numerical metrics mandated by global health funders today not only have the power to determine
which interventions are successes, which are failures, which will be funded,
and which will not, but they also carry the political clout to determine who
will get reelected to office, who will be promoted to chief medical director
of a hospital, and who will win a government contract. Metrics, in other
words, carry a certain political efficacy in the wake of their health impacts.
This political efficacy does not emerge as an artifact of numerical neutrality.
I argue that the political efficacy of metrics works as a condition of their
production, a mandate built into their collection, and ultimately a constitutive basis for their meaning. In this way the numbers matter in ways that
far exceed the accounting exercises of global health.

The entanglements of politics and metrics productivity result from a
push for numerical proof of effectiveness that determines not only who is
counted but also how health care is delivered — in other words, determining which women are metrically seen and which are not. New regimes of
global health accountability in maternal health thus create problematic alliances among politicians, states, and fiscal institutions that encourage these
states to organize themselves as recipient nations in and around problems
concerning not health per se but numbers meant to represent health. When
local sovereignty — local political authority grounded in territory — is tethered to the numbers games that arrive with global health grant-giving organizations, practices of accountability, cost efficiency, and translatability can
create perverse incentives for local politicians.

Linking Numbers and Dollars

Since the election of its current governor in early 2009 — an election that
was itself craftily managed around a contestation of numbers[3] — this southwestern Nigerian state government has in many ways organized itself
around agendas set by the United Nations, the World Health Organization
(WHO), and other leading international health organizations. Built in 2010,
the Hospital for Mothers and Children (HMC), with its bright green roofs,
thick cement walls, and rooms equipped with hospital gadgetry dating

from a few years to a few decades old, is the crowning achievement of the state's HMHB program, the governor's specific response to a World Bank study, the 2008 Nigeria Demographic and Health Survey (NDHS).

The NDHS study found that this Nigerian state was one of the furthest from reaching the United Nation's Millennium Development Goal 5,[4] which aimed to improve maternal health by reducing maternal deaths to three quarters of the rate in 1990 by 2015 and achieving universal access to reproductive health. Focused on increasing the number of women who give birth in approved health facilities with skilled birth attendants, HMHB now offers free biomedical health care to all pregnant women and children under five. The governor, the commissioner of health, and several international agencies have gathered enough preliminary quantitative evidence to make the claim that because of the steps they have taken their state will be one of very few places in sub-Saharan Africa to succeed in reaching Goal 5. The evidence for this claim relies primarily on a study conducted over a twelve-month period starting in June 2012 which found that the maternal mortality rate, originally estimated at 545 deaths per 100,000 live births in the 2008 NDHS, had been reduced to 253, a more than 50 percent reduction.

Today the government presents HMHB as a comprehensive approach to maternal and child health care. It is modeled as a four-tiered health system, with HMC in the state's capital city meant to be a quaternary referral hospital for especially challenging cases coming from more rurally situated primary care centers. Within the state a local government area or "county" near the capital served as the pilot region for the program. There efforts to implement HMHB resulted in the transformation or, in some cases, abandonment of small clinics that previously saw all types of patients but were sorely neglected. This was done to make way for HMHB basic health centers and comprehensive health centers. These centers now serve as primary and secondary care centers, respectively, for pregnant women and children under five only. General hospitals are tertiary care centers that can be utilized by all, but they are slightly less accessible to rural populations. Basic health centers are entirely run by nurses and midwives who attend normal vaginal deliveries independently. If a doctor is needed to manage hypertension or diabetes in pregnancy, for example, the woman is transferred to a comprehensive health center or general hospital. If a cesarean section is called for, she is transferred to HMC. Women who register their pregnancies early enough at a basic health center are supposed to get cell phones so they can keep in touch with their "health ranger," a community health worker who is assigned to regularly visit them in their homes and respond to any of their health concerns.

The rolling out of the HMHB program represents more than a response by health planners to health concerns that were not previously being met in maternal health care. HMHB represents the outcome of a new alliance in the structures of funding for global health provisions. While government programs have long been dominated by global health agendas that link monetary resources to acceptance of externally designed models for programming, how this process continues today through various forms of counting is worth exploring.

Less than two years after the launch of HMHB, this particular state became the recipient of a $60 million health investment loan from the World Bank. This is not entirely surprising since it was the World Bank that sponsored the NDHS, the study that motivated the creation of HMHB in the first place. The program, having gained international recognition, has since received additional grants from the Ford Foundation and the Bill and Melinda Gates Foundation. Not all of these are loans, but all of the funding is portrayed as needed by the state government's Ministry of Health to solve the problem of maternal mortality. Without the financial aid, certain health care resources and programs might not exist.

The links between quantitative health statistics and international agency financial support having been established, the government naturally seeks to keep the grant money flowing in by continuing to supply the data needed to affirm the utility and impact of this money. This is even more explicitly demonstrated beyond the work of maternal health. On a fall 2011 visit to Nigeria, Bill Gates met with President Goodluck Jonathan to discuss the country's commitment to ending polio. As a result of this visit the Gates Foundation in partnership with the Nigerian Governor's Forum launched the Governor's Immunization Leadership Challenge. The initiative, lasting the twelve calendar months of 2012, was aimed at eradicating new cases of polio from Nigeria by the end of 2012, and an award for the states that immunized the most babies was set at $500,000 with the promise of an additional $250,000 if the government of the winning states made a matching contribution. The funds, potentially $1 million in total, were to be put toward further improving health care and delivery in the winning states. Of the six states that emerged as winners in early 2013, the state that had coincidently recently launched the HMHB initiative came in first with the highest recorded rates of polio vaccination in Nigeria.

The achievement was highly publicized by the state government and local newspapers in a year that coincided with the state election in which the current governor was up for reelection. A press release in late 2012 announced the state's lead in the race to eradicate polio according to the Gates Foundation's third-quarter assessment, which estimated its immunization coverage at 85 percent. When the winners were announced early in the following year, several local and national news organizations reported on the state's success, applauding its governor as the best performing governor in the country. Like winning the global health Olympics, this odd strategy of mixing the language of fiscal gaming with real program needs in polio eradication reflected a healthy dose of market-oriented global health planning; not only were there winners and losers in the game of keeping lives healthy, but the strategy also involved shifting some fiscal responsibility back onto the recipient state. The governor himself was quoted as saying, "Winning the 2012 Bill and Melinda Gates Polio Challenge was an added impetus to pursue more aggressive health care projects in the state."[5]

In Nigeria the patterns of funding and accountability seen in the race to stop polio have spilled over into maternal and child health efforts. I attended a meeting between high-level state government officials and representatives from Family Health Organization, a Nigerian nongovernmental organization chosen by the Gates Foundation to implement the Immunization Leadership Challenge and ensure proper usage of the contest winnings. The deputy director of Family Health Organization and local grants manager of the Immunization Leadership Challenge opened the meeting by saying, "I'm sure that we all know that [this] state was overall first in Nigeria in the organization's challenge . . . so our mission here is to ensure that that first position is sustained, to maintain it." Another representative from Family Health Organization chimed in, "The world will say that [this] state emerged as the best not by [a] fluke but by our action and our proactive activities."

The rest of the meeting was dedicated to detailing how the contest winnings would be used for the HMHB program, the hope being to identify gaps and challenges that the money could be used to address. While the principal problem discussed was the fact that women still frequent church-based birthing centers and traditional birth attendants (TBAS) rather than going to free government-sponsored clinics, the meeting attendees agreed that money should go to scaling up the HMHB program to the seventeen other local government areas in the state. One high-level government official explained, "If we improve facilities, we can improve facility deliveries by 20 to 30 percent, . . . [and] TBAS will naturally phase out." Caught up in the fervor of success that was mapped out in the polio contest, these health care officials saw opportunities to generate even more success in their work in maternal and child health care. Rather than orient themselves toward the particularities of a pressing local problem, they sought to align themselves with more easily quantifiable goals.

What is interesting about this case is how the numbers, once produced in the polio effort and later in the maternal health effort, became instruments for political mobility and economic advancement. The instance of the Gates Foundation Immunization Leadership Challenge and the supervening events in this state tied successful hospital and clinic statistics to the problem of securing government resources to do any work at all. The numbers here represented more than simple metrics to help decide which interventions worked and which did not; they became indices of successful governance because they were the conduit for securing more aid. Let us not forget that the official name of the contest was the *Governor's* Immunization *Leadership* Challenge. The statistics used in the polio campaign and the Gates Foundation resources became quickly visible not just in WHO Millennium Development Goals status reports and Gates Foundation annual letters but also in the local state's election campaigns, helping voters to discern good leaders from bad ones. The problem with the increasing reliance on numbers, however, is that once they are circulating in this political way, it becomes difficult to question them. Their power multiplies.

Affirming the intertwining of local politics with what is now largely NGO-based global health aid, Bill Gates and Aliko Dangote, Nigeria's own multibillionaire (in U.S. dollars), have joined forces to facilitate a $50 million Japan International Cooperation Agency loan to Nigeria with the aim of "fighting" polio. On the same visit to Nigeria in which the loan was announced, Gates's fourth in a series of visits related to polio eradication, President Jonathan recognized his assistance to the country by awarding him the second highest Nigerian national honor, Commander of the Federal Republic. This is an award that the late celebrated Nigerian author Chinua Achebe declined twice, citing unaddressed rampant government corruption. With so many international dollars at stake, it is no wonder that maintaining and managing "the numbers" is seen as a primary task of politicians. The specifics of how this is accomplished are important to track, as the consequences for the health of those who are not counted are potentially devastating.

The Governor's Brainchild: The Stakes beyond Health

International donor reliance on accountability by way of metrics creates perverse incentives for individuals in recipient countries to produce numbers in specific ways and often in ways that attend more to political than health goals. Those who stand to gain politically if they can produce evidence of a successful intervention are likely to gain the most if the numbers are good.

The HMHB initiative has brought millions of dollars into the state, boosting the economy and creating jobs for health care workers and government subcontractors. While one might easily recognize the positive value of these changes, the fact that the work holding them together is so focused on accountability assessed exclusively with numbers can also be problematic, as Wendland (this volume) has shown. Everyone, from patients to doctors and government officials, becomes complicit in the push to produce and also exhibit good data, that is, data that show improvement. Bad data, data that might show weakness in the system, are frequently discounted or kept invisible. Following Erikson (2012: 379; this volume), I am concerned with how the business of global health creates pressure for "death data to 'go missing,'" as seen in Blessing's story. At the same time, Western-African partnerships differentially affect individuals in recipient countries; some are able to capitalize on incoming sources of funding, while others do not share in the spoils (Crane 2010b, 2013; Kalofonos 2014). Often HMHB program doctors feel constrained and unable to care for their patients in the way they think best. Before returning to this group of actors, I focus here on those whose fates and fortunes appear to be most obviously tied to the success of the program.

Though maternal mortality does not appear among Nigeria's top ten causes of death (Institute for Health Metrics and Evaluation 2013), it has changed the political landscape of this state considerably. The governor, previously a practicing physician, ran on a platform that featured his health-related achievements and was reelected in 2012. He is the first governor to win a second term in this state. Two of the cabinet members who were reappointed, one of whom is the commissioner of health, are also medical doctors. Both the governor and the commissioner of health travel across the globe, presenting lectures on the success of the HMHB program at conferences in places ranging from Washington, DC to Beijing. Health, or at least the state's claim to fame in global health communities, dominates local politics and possibilities of upward socioeconomic mobility.

This statewide focus on health is not lost on the citizens of this state, who refer to HMC and the HMHB program as "the governor's brainchild." Patients associate the care they receive at the hospital with the governor and the state's prosperity. One woman proudly exclaimed, in response to a question about why she chose to have her child at HMC, "This place is our [governor]'s, [this] state [governor]'s. It belongs to everybody!" Patients and their family members often enthusiastically support the hospital, rejoicing in its reported successes. The governor and his wife were at this time wildly popular, drawing considerable attention at even the sight of their motorcade.

Many of the doctors I spoke to at HMC also associate the HMHB program and health care with the potential for political achievement. When asked what field they wanted to go into after finishing their intern year, the most common answer was "politics." Doctors aspire to complete a residency, which is not actually a requirement to practice in Nigeria, or a master's degree in business administration or public health from an overseas university as a means of rising up the medical ladder and, subsequently, the political ladder. The current commissioner of health was previously the chief medical director of a hospital before obtaining a foreign degree and being appointed to office.

Hopes of benefiting from the success of the HMHB program did not end with doctors. Over lunch the commissioner of health's driver, Taiwo, told me he had been working for the ministry for ten years, but, he assured me, the present commissioner had been his "best boss." Taiwo said he had learned so much from the commissioner and that the commissioner made it a point of taking care of his employees. "We are all praying for them to nominate him to the federal office. Maybe Goodluck Jonathan will just pick him [to be the nation's minister of health], and we will all just go with him to Abuja!"

With all the political and economic capital garnered by HMHB, individuals and private companies that previously had little to do with health or health care have also begun to shift their focus to health in order to win government contracts and profit from the HMHB program rollout. I spent one afternoon with the commissioner of health as he sifted through a foot-high stack of mail. There were proposals from both NGOs and private companies to take part in the HMHB program. One man wrote to request more money for payment on the gas station that the government acquired for the building of a second HMC in another town. Another requested the balance of the money owed for the replacement of the roof at the HMC in the state's capital. Apparently 600 million Naira was owed and only 3 million Naira was paid by the government (the exchange rate was then roughly US$1 to 160 Naira). Other companies wrote proposals to provide the new hospitals with everything from flat screen TVs to continuing education seminars for staff.

The HMHB program has become woven into politics almost as if it were itself a new branch or institutional form of governance in this region. The careers of many individuals are contingent on the continued success of the program; that is, they are perpetuated by the production of specific kinds of data to show that the program has done what it set out to do: reduce maternal mortality rates, keeping more mothers and children alive than was previously possible. And this is what the quantitative data collected are effective at doing. With so much relying on the state's maternal mortality rates, it is not surprising that everyone becomes complicit in projecting a successful HMHB program.

The chief medical director of HMC, Dr. Adetunde, is not alone in wanting to discount Blessing's death. Erikson (2012: 373) reminds us that in the global health business, "whether statistics are accurate enough to improve health is less important than whether statistics are performed and work to enable economic systems." Statistics "enable other things of value, like gainful employment and profit-making" (373). These new regimes of data production act as technologies of governance that contribute to a new global sovereignty but do not always align with local needs.

It might be argued that this restructuring in terms of finance and implementation through HMHB (and other programs inspired by the Millennium Development Goals in other regions of other countries) has made such a big difference that it does merit recognition as a Millennium Development Goal 5 success. But what kinds of numbers must be in circulation for this to be the case? If numbers that show positive outcomes become compulsory for a developing region's success in the eyes of the donors who keep programs in nations like Nigeria alive, little room is left for questioning the numbers or how they are collected and become known. Yet when numbers become essential to local political and economic success—as I illustrated with the governor's popularity, several doctors' aspirations, and private business contract winners—it becomes important to ask how the numbers must change, how they must be produced, and what purposes they must serve far beyond the problems of women like Blessing.

Limited Possibilities for Care

A close analysis of clinical encounters in HMHB hospitals reveals how aid industry mandates to collect data as "proof of success" force individuals to perform data in a way that can be both constraining for doctors and detrimental to patients. As Adams (2013a: 55) notes, the turn in global health communities toward an insistence on numerical data leads to a "shift in priorities in caregiving practices in public health such that 'people [no longer] come first'" because the demand for quantitative results often means abstracting clinical care from the social relationships on which these results depend. Even the very act of gathering data can affect the ways data collectors are oriented toward and interact with patients. Biruk (2012: 348) has demonstrated in her work on AIDS research in Malawi that the precise way in which studies demand data be collected manifests in the "gestures, comportments, habits, and interactions of fieldworkers and research subjects." Focusing on relationships between caregivers and HIV patients, Kalofonos (2014) tracks how the rapid and technical HIV scale-up in Mozambique narrowed conceptions of what constitutes care to strictly clinically oriented work, leaving out other, less technical forms of care—domestic chores or prayer, for example. Here I pay attention to both data and care by exploring how the possibilities for caregiving, a supposed primary goal of global health, are undermined by the need to "perform data" (Erikson 2012) and be accountable to both overseas funding sources and local political agendas.

In 2010 the state House Assembly members unanimously signed into law a confidential maternal death audit bill. Recognizing that before the start of HMHB only 16 percent of women delivered in health facilities, the law is designed to better track maternal deaths in the state. It notes that when a woman dies, a relative must report the death within forty-eight hours, irrespective of where the death occurred. Failure to do so violates the law and will incur jail time and/or fines. There are no punitive measures for reporting. The law thus makes reporting both more important and more problematic than ever before.

At a House Assembly meeting in which the origins of the law were presented to legislators visiting from another state, the medical director of one of the HMHB hospitals spoke, emphasizing the importance of confidentiality. "The law goes a long way in protecting the confidentiality of the informant." He later added, "No name, no shame, no blame." At the same time, the government has clear motives for the law beyond merely keeping count. Another high-level government official said, "[The new law] laid the foundations for the accurate measurement and tracking of maternal deaths in the state upon which policy formulations can be based." With data on where maternal deaths happen outside of HMHB hospitals and clinics, the government can make decisions about where women will be allowed to give birth.

Perhaps because the politics matter so much to local participants in HMHB, and because there is so much riding on the production of the right kinds of numbers in the program, the state government has taken steps to produce its own data. Rather than rely on outside agencies like the World Bank to perform epidemiological studies related to maternal and child health, the state government now seeks to take data collection into its own hands. The new law gives the appearance of producing more reliable data in order to prove that the in-hospital HMHB program is working (which is important to international donors). In actuality production of numbers through this law is not without contestation, as we have seen in the case of Blessing. The demand for data that can be used to prove the success of HMHB has not only changed the way women receive care (in ways that are not always beneficial to the patients); it has also constrained the way doctors are allowed to practice.

The day after Eid, the feast at the end of the Muslim holy month of Ramadan and a federal holiday in Nigeria, a man named Sunday approached Dr. Olamide, the chief medical director of the newly built HMC in his town. Sunday explained that his wife, Funmi, needed to be seen urgently. That morning she had started coughing, and her sutures from the cesarean section she had the week before had opened up. He claimed that nobody would attend to her in the emergency department. Dr. Olamide told Sunday to go back to the emergency department and that the nurses there would help him. When, a few minutes later, Dr. Olamide noticed that Sunday was still standing with Funmi in the hall outside the emergency room without being seen, he charged down the hall toward the two of them and ordered them to enter the emergency room. He told Funmi that she shouldn't be moving about and that she should have a seat.

He took Sunday to the card registration office and then stormed back into the emergency room, flinging reprimands at the nurse, who was tending to another patient. "Now you will be wondering why patients beat you guys up!" he shouted in Yoruba, referring to an incident in which a nurse had been assaulted by the father of a pediatric patient who had died at the HMC in another town. "Why was this patient not seen? This is an emergency!"

He ushered Funmi into a makeshift examination "room" in the corner of the emergency room, surrounded the bed with blue cloth dividers, and asked her to lie down. Pulling up her top, we were all shocked to see a loop of Funmi's bowels protruding from the incision in her abdomen. Dr. Olamide yelled for other doctors to come help place an IV, start her on antibiotics, draw blood to be cross-matched in preparation for surgery, and cover the exposed intestines with sterile gauze. Funmi lay on the bed, becoming more terrified with every exclamation from Dr. Olamide.

In the aftermath I talked to everyone involved in the incident: Funmi, the nurse, the emergency room intern, and Dr. Olamide. When I asked Funmi what happened, she explained that she had had a cough. That morning when she was coughing, her belly had burst open. She said she hadn't told anyone in the emergency room that her insides had broken through her skin because no one had asked. She told them only that she wanted to see a doctor. Both the nurse and the intern said they didn't know that Funmi had a burst abdomen and that they were just following protocol. Before even being seen by a nurse, a patient is normally expected to go to hospital registration to get a registration card and casebook. The casebook contains the patient's medical history, and she cannot be seen without it. Detailed records must be taken at the start of every patient encounter. Once the casebook is obtained, a nurse can see the patient, followed by a doctor.

While these expectations for record-keeping protocol might seem commonplace and even reassuring to the outsider, especially if one is familiar with hospitals in wealthier countries, one wonders why emergency room protocols would not have streamlined the process for a case like Funmi's. The dedication to record-keeping outweighed a dedication to the patient so that there was no room for improvising on behalf of the patient even in her pressing medical circumstances. This is why the chief medical director

Cultural problem surrounding data

was furious. He felt that Funmi and her husband looked anxious enough that a nurse should have asked her what was wrong. Had the nurse done this, he explained to me, she would have known that it was an emergency and that protocol did not need to be followed. But the worry is that for hospitals like those in the HMHB program, where staff are trained to consider the urgency of recording data on patients to be just as important as attending to their health needs, these record-keeping operations can sometimes get in the way of appropriate care.

Funmi's burst abdomen was eventually treated, but during the time that she and her husband spent trying to navigate the hospital's record-keeping operations, her internal organs had been exposed unnecessarily to infection. Dr. Olamide was clear that in cases like this, keeping records should not be the priority. Yet possibilities for successful clinical care are sometimes impeded by the compulsion to produce data. At the same time, it is this compulsion to produce data for the HMHB program that is vital to the survival of not only hospitals but also careers like his.

It is true that demands for accountability can structure and shape how medicine gets practiced in most places in the world and particularly in hospitals. One might find oversight like this in any emergency ward in any country. However, in this state the overwhelming presence of the HMHB program (and its need to prove its success in order to ensure continued funding) became a particularly strong structuring force in determining how clinical care was carried out, how triage was determined, and how patients were made visible or invisible. One wonders how Funmi's case would have been recorded had she died. So much effort had been made to get her case on the ledger. Would she have been recorded as a failure on the part of the hospital, or would she not have been recorded at all, seen as a patient who came to the clinic too late and beyond the reach of those delivering care?

Younger doctors, not yet caught up in HMHB propaganda, were particularly vocal about the conflicts of interest inherent in the program. They expressed discontent with their supervisors' political pandering at the expense of patient well-being. They considered such pandering a form of "politics" in the sense that they suspected their supervisors were depending on the success of HMHB for personal gain and thus to become potential candidates for promotion. Many also recognized that these successes depended on a process of data collection that was at odds with the notion of best practices that they had been taught in medical school. Contestation between caregivers was often aroused by the explicit perception that decisions were being made on the basis of the need for certain kinds of numbers and certain kinds of outcomes.

One young doctor at the HMC ranted about Dr. Olamide on the morning after his call, "I don't like the way the [chief medical director] talks to me." I spent the night on call with him, following him as he made rounds on the patients in the antenatal, postnatal, and delivery wards. During down time we watched a news program in Chinese in the doctors' lounge while we waited for the nurses to come calling with patient complaints. Just before midnight a woman arrived at the hospital with the complaint that her water broke. As she was only twenty-six weeks pregnant, the young doctor thought this was unlikely, but he performed a vaginal exam and assessed the woman for signs of early labor, as he had been taught to do. The vaginal exam showed that the opening to her uterus, her cervix, was closed and there was no sign of her water breaking. He was all set to discharge her when he received a call from Dr. Olamide, who, although he had not seen the patient, told him to admit her anyway. The young doctor was surprised by this demand. Women who were not yet in labor and who were not otherwise in distress would normally be sent home. Still the young doctor admitted her, but not without complaining to everyone who would listen. When the next team of doctors came to relieve him the following morning, he recounted the story for them. The three other doctors groaned in support.

> "If they want us to be admitting patients like this, we will admit everyone and the whole hospital will be full, and then when an eclamptic case [a potentially deadly obstetric emergency] comes, we will have to turn them away. That's what we will start doing."
>
> Another doctor shrugged in agreement.
>
> "It's all political," yet another added.

It is not entirely clear why Dr. Olamide insisted that the young doctor admit this patient in particular. While Dr. Olamide was confident that he had made a medically warranted decision, the younger doctors were convinced that there were other factors at play. Was Dr. Olamide's desire to admit the potentially unproblematic case built on his desire for better statistics, or was he motivated by something entirely different—VIP treatment for friends of high-level politicians, for example? Everyone working in maternal care cares immensely about successful outcomes for patients,

But sometimes when outcomes can be used as political ammunition, strategies for admission, triage, and counting can become very confusing. Again, we cannot be sure why the woman was admitted, but it is important to consider seriously the sentiments of the young doctor and his colleagues. They were frustrated because they felt that Dr. Olamide's politics had trumped their own sense of best medical practices. They had learned that a woman pregnant for twenty-six weeks with a closed cervix and no other complaints should be sent home. Admitting this woman could potentially displace a later urgent care patient at greater risk of dying.

The young doctors in the hospitals that I visited often talked about how the relationship between the hospital, the HMHB initiative, and the government's office was constraining their medical decisions in ways that were not necessarily medically justifiable. The chief medical director, the commissioner of health, and even the governor could veto any one of their decisions at any time, and they lived with the persistent fear that they would be chastised for their decisions despite the medical basis for them. Even with set protocols, doctors found that certain situations and certain patients called for special attention; these tactics were usually related to processes unknown to them, but that most assumed they were based on politics is significant.

The grievances among doctors revealed discord in how the HMHB program sought to ensure the visibility of its own success. They raise questions about the regime of data productivity, in which HMHB is a site not only for maternal care but also for political exigencies. In situations like the one the young doctor found himself in, caregivers become acutely aware that it is impossible to be neutral when it comes to the care the hospital provides and subsequently the numerical data it produces—or worse, that doctors shouldn't rely solely on their own medical opinion. Recognizing that the numbers that HMHB strives to produce are not neutral, caregivers feel trapped, constrained in the care they give by a political vision and global processes that are beyond their control.

Conclusion

The story of the HMHB program in southwestern Nigeria is a novel instance of an often-told story in global health; think of the ways structural adjustment and vertical aid programs undermine state sovereignty and local practices of health care (Farmer 2001; Foley 2009; Kalofonos 2014;

Keshavjee 2014; Pfeiffer and Chapman 2010; Watts 1994). Here, however, the state gains its economic power through interactions with global health agencies. Rather than a state increasingly confined to progressively smaller spheres of influence and power as international health donor agencies restructure themselves into private enterprises and work directly with local hospitals, the regional government works *with* multilateral development agencies and not-for-profit private grant-making foundations to ensure its own survival. The shell of the state remains in the figures of local health actors who aspire to become ministers, politicians, and leaders who will govern by way of the demands set by the agendas of international donors.

Development aid still figures prominently in the governance of places and people in this region. Because of the ways this aid is tied to productivity and success, the work of health development increasingly relies on numbers to not only guide but also to give support to specific health activities. The demand for numerical proficiency and certain kinds of success-showing numbers eventually forms a sort of governance or global sovereignty over both clinical practices and political processes. That is, on their way to affecting health outcomes, the numbers have a way of producing political effects that exceed the mere production of numerical facts. This is not simply a case of neutral numbers falling into the wrong hands. The numbers themselves are produced and performed in ways that imbue them with political efficacy. But the work they do — a result of the work done to produce them — can have real consequences for both how patients are treated and who wins elections.

I am not suggesting that the call for accountability underlying the steadily growing push for a universal metrics in global health is necessarily a bad thing (Adams 2013a). However, when the numbers go unquestioned, when they are allowed to stand for much more than they were originally intended to measure and become instruments of political aggrandizement, we should be wary. Numbers are seductive in their seamless utility. They turn complicated, messy local realities into manageable, translatable, comparable figures. However, these same qualities give the increasing primacy of numbers in global health an ominous power that can elide clinical realities, compromise care, and hide some kinds of death.

As many of the authors in this volume demonstrate, relying only on numbers to create global health agendas has the potential for detrimental effects. The HMHB program demonstrates that numbers are not only hard to collect in an unbiased manner but may not accurately describe a situation, as was the case for the uncounted woman, Blessing. At every level of data production, efforts to direct flows of money and political power weaken claims to objectivity. The point is this: there is no such thing as objectivity in this sort of situation. There are only numbers and politics. Recognizing how these work as well as when and how they don't is more important than ever. When doing global health means doing global health *research*, certain health solutions and health practices that cannot be measured numerically are left out. Blessing was uncounted because she was marked as dying in transit and her death would have marred the hospital's claim to success. Money is spent on building more government health facilities rather than negotiating solutions with traditional birth attendants or church-based facilities because the numbers of women who attend government health facilities can be more easily counted and monitored. Meanwhile up to 80 percent of women in much of Nigeria still deliver outside of a hospital or clinic. The care they get is unquantifiable by global health standards and thus remains unaccounted for.

My hope in presenting cases like this is that questions about how we produce numbers and demonstrate accountability will be more carefully considered, particularly as the global health industry continues to mandate that we use numbers-based ways of knowing the world in relation to a diverse and complex set of health problems and situations. Rather paradoxically numerical standards for effectiveness can sometimes create incentives for recipient countries and organizations to "perform good data" in ways that limit potentially productive possibilities for health care.

Notes

1. In order to protect confidentiality, I use pseudonyms for most of the people and organizations mentioned. The only exceptions to this rule are well-known figures and institutions whose actions are widely published, including Bill Gates, the Bill and Melinda Gates Foundation, Nigerian president Goodluck Jonathan, Aliko Dangote, the Japan International Cooperation Agency, the Ford Foundation, WHO, and the World Bank.

2. While fieldwork was completed in Nigeria over three months during the summer of 2013, conversations with informants extended into the next year through phone, email, and social media. Funding was provided by a grant from the Bixby Center for Population, Health, and Sustainability at the University of California, Berkeley School of Public Health.

3. The present governor actually originally lost the April 2007 elections but then

contested the results in a nonpartisan election petitions tribunal. The tribunal found irregularities in the 2007 election, putting the current governor in office in 2008. The national Court of Appeals in Benin subsequently unanimously upheld the results of the state election petitions tribunal.

4. According to the 2008 NDHS, this state had the lowest rate of births delivered in a health facility (49.2 percent) and assisted by a skilled provider (50.5 percent). The rates for the other five states in southwest Nigeria ranged from 67.1 to 85.1 percent and 71.8 to 89.2 percent, respectively.

5. Johnson 2013; Sodiq Oyeleke, "Polio Award, an Invitation to Do More — Mimiko," *Punch*, November 13, 2013, accessed July 9, 2015, http://www.punchng.com/?s=polio +award.

PART II. METRICS POLITICS

4 · THE POWER OF DATA Global Malaria Governance
and the Senegalese Data Retention Strike MARLEE TICHENOR

From July 2010 until March 2013 members of two Senegalese health worker unions followed a *mot d'ordre* to withhold routine patient data from the central Ministry of Health while continuing to perform their duties as health care providers. This strike was meant to impact their working conditions, but they also wanted to use the strike as a way to bring light to health care resource distribution inequality across the country. Although the official statement on the strike was that it was appealing solely to the Senegalese government, some union members made it clear to me that the union convergence leadership was also aware that by withholding health data they were also undermining the relationship between Senegal and the international aid community. Current forms of global health funding require tightly regulated evidence, proving to the international aid community that their aid has real impact on the local situation, to justify supporting health programs in the Global South. In the public health fight against malaria in Senegal, the data retention strike seriously threatened the country's ability to get funding from the Global Fund to Fight AIDS, Tuberculosis, and Malaria for the next funding cycle, in 2013. As such, the strike demonstrates that regular and precise production of local health data plays a key role in the global enterprise. By striking in this way, health workers appealed not only to the national leadership but also to a distinctly global community for recognition of their rights.

If the new global sovereign is a "flexible assemblage of data production, number crunching, and scale-up profit sourcing that . . . orchestrates biopolitical health interventions so that they work within capitalism's terms and limits" (Adams: chapter 1, this volume), then it is important to consider how contemporary regimes of governance are perhaps built upon global health inventions of measurement in very particular ways. As Wendland shows in her Malawian case study in this volume, health metrics are often abstracted and estimated explicitly to be compared in regional and global contexts, and those metrics, when showing "success" in attacking specific health indicators, are then used to legitimize local governments. The tension created by the data retention strike in Senegal illuminates the power of metrics in efforts to determine "success" in the fight against malaria and in their absence for three years, the strike also illuminates the necessity of such data for Senegal's malaria governance sector to survive.

According to some scholars (Cooper 1997; Ferguson 1994), many governments in sub-Saharan Africa have been configured since independence to participate in markets of development aid. In this context the metrics produced about a country's health profile are tied to what kind of aid that country can receive and its ability to support its own health system. In an era of the Millennium Development Goals, the measurement of a country's need for development aid is tied to that country's likelihood—or rather unlikelihood—of reaching those goals. In turn, the production of the data required to measure national neediness can be understood as a component of the performance of not just politics (as Oni-Orisan notes, this volume) but also the performance of citizenship.

In Senegal there is a rich history of labor as a crucial part of citizenship even before the country's independence from France in 1960. In the health sector, as Tousignant (2013: 97) shows, Senegalese pharmacists have expressed their own citizenship through their performance as "guarantors of quality" of pharmaceuticals. In the context of the health data retention strike, their labor not only as health workers but also as data producers played a key role in their performance of citizenship. Indeed, the striking health workers understood that the Senegalese Ministry of Health and its partners needed their routine data in order to properly manage and organize public health initiatives. A representative of the union convergence leadership told me that health workers are exceptional sorts of workers: they must have access to rights and protections like any other union worker, but they also have a "moral obligation to provide care to others, bound as [they] are by the Hippocratic Oath." The leadership of the union convergence chose to strike by retaining information because they felt it was a more "humanistic" approach to sway the national government; they would continue to provide care and fulfill the most pressing moral obligation, but they could simultaneously withhold something of value from the government, knowing full well that this was a place of political leverage.

Current global health governance can be divided into two regimes: *global health security* and *humanitarian biomedicine*. Andrew Lakoff (2010) argues that global health security focuses on "emerging infectious diseases," like SARS or influenzas, that come from the Global South and threaten the health of populations in the Global North. Global health security is focused on preparation and the *anticipation* of large-scale pandemics. Humanitarian biomedicine, however, is focused on diseases that primarily impact poorer nations, putting the "suffering individual" at the center of its framework and creating "apolitical" networks among researchers, local health workers, private industry, and activists. At work in this regime is the notion that in order to get health care to individuals, "intervention is seen as necessary where public health infrastructure at the nation-state level is in poor condition or non-existent" (61).

In Senegal the large-scale management of malaria through the National Malaria Control Program emerges at the intersection of these two regimes of global health. The disease impacts primarily vulnerable populations in the Global South, but malaria is hardly a "neglected disease." Research and development for malaria has increased exponentially in the past couple decades, and it is recognized as one of the Big Three of global health (along with HIV/AIDS and tuberculosis), which receive the largest amount of funds allocated for global health. With the inclusion of the reduction of malaria morbidity and mortality as a Millennium Development Goal in 2000, the number of projects and funding for combating the disease at least quadrupled in the past two decades (Roll Back Malaria Partnership

2010).[1] This effort led to the creation in 1998 of an international orchestrating body called the Roll Back Malaria Partnership (RBM) to organize the highly heterogeneous network of partners combating the disease and to the creation of donor entities like the Global Fund in 2002 and USAID's President's Malaria Initiative (PMI) in 2006.

Despite the fact that malaria has plagued human populations, by some estimates (Shah 2010) for hundreds of millennia, the disease has come to be defined as an object of humanitarian urgency, particularly with regard to the surveillance of emerging resistance to artemisinin, the drug currently recommended by the World Health Organization (WHO) to treat uncomplicated forms of malaria. Surveillance has become a key tool in the humanitarian fight against the disease, and locally produced health data of all kinds have become crucial to this effort. These data include: what pharmaceuticals are administered and in what dosages; how often patients come in; how long their symptoms last; whether they experience side effects to the pharmaceuticals; and the results from laboratory testing, if available. It is precisely through an examination of the role of locally produced health data (and the labor required to produce them) that we can come to understand the complicated relationship between local actors and the vast assemblage of organizations and funders that constitute the regulatory body of global malaria governance.

Unlike the case of Indonesia's refusal to share H5N1 virus samples with the international community in 2007, the Senegalese health worker data retention strike was not condoned by the Senegalese state.[2] These two cases are different in many key ways, but they both bring into focus the value of locally produced data and power relations that are often presented as neutral among the many different scales of the global health fight against malaria, from the level of the community health worker to those of the academic researcher and the grant auditor. Appealing both to national representation and global representation and astutely discerning the importance of the data they produce on a local level, striking health union members also highlight the ways that surveillance and regulation are necessary for their government's participation in a global market through global malaria governance. They make explicit the implicit reciprocal trade relationship of data for funding in the global health fight against the disease.

The Senegalese Health System and
the Global Fight against Malaria

In 1992 Senegal implemented the Bamako Initiative in its national health system, standardizing health management and monitoring throughout the country. The Bamako Initiative sought to increase accessibility to health care through the decentralization of the national system, giving more autonomy to individual health posts, centers, and hospitals.[3] Since its establishment, different partners in the malaria world have pointed out that the decentralization of the health system has led to an inconsistency of approaches to combating the disease and to a particular oversight in and around addressing preventative measures (National Malaria Control Program of Senegal [NMCP] 2001).

Soon after the Bamako Initiative was implemented, the National Malaria Control Program was established within the Ministry of Health in 1995. In 1999 Senegal became a part of the Roll Back Malaria Partnership (set up as a partnership between the WHO, the United Nations Children's Fund, the United Nations Development Program, and the World Bank), which has the goal of harmonizing the multiple efforts to combat the disease. The proliferation of funds and organizations around combating malaria in Senegal has had many effects, including the use of malaria control efforts to pilot health care initiatives in general in the country (such as the monitoring of pharmaceutical quality and side effects). Most striking, it has led to a further fragmentation of the ways that health care is managed from above in Senegal.

With the decentralization of public health that came with the Bamako Initiative, communities became financially responsible for many parts of the health system, including the building and maintenance of health facilities and the salaries of local health workers. In rural areas of Senegal (including the southeast region of Kédougou, which has one of the highest malaria transmission rates in the country) much of the funding for community health infrastructure and human resources came from remittances of those community members who had gone to work in one of the *grandes villes* in the region or in Europe. The attempt to make these health systems self-sustaining ultimately undermined their viability. The local community health committee has to approve funding of different initiatives, including the hiring and training of community members to become health workers. However, as an NMCP representative informed me, often in these rural health districts a community will invest in the training of a local health worker who will work in the region for a short while before using that training to emigrate to a *grande ville* or out of the country. In this context, health facilities in rural regions, more often than not, have extremely limited access to equipment, experience frequent ruptures in essential medicines, and lack sufficiently trained health workers. Still, the demands made on these people to produce accountability data remains steady.

The international web of public and private funders and public and private interveners demands that the Senegalese NMCP, and the NMCPs of other countries receiving international malaria funding, become institutions of accountability. In efforts to represent the needs of their own populations to the international community, these agencies must deploy people to generate data in very specific forms (see Biruk 2012). Despite the fact that the kinds of data that these organizations demand are sometimes impossible to come by and always already not neutral, the NMCP must mediate among a variety of different interests in order to secure funding for malaria programs; these result in mediated policies that trickle down to the workers at the bottom of the health care hierarchy—that is, to those who collect the data. The role of health workers in this web of accountability becomes extremely clear with the data retention strike, much to the frustration of many of those working at and with the NMCP. Thus, health workers themselves recognize their responsibility to the regime of accountability, and the dissenting union opinion has been to remind the union convergence at large that that they need to fulfill that role for the good of the national health system in general (Secretariat du Comité Central du PIT 2011).

The 2010–2013 Health Worker Data Retention Strike

In July 2010 a convergence of two health worker unions, the Syndicat Unique des Travailleurs de la Santé et de l'Action Sociale (SUTSAS) and the Syndicat Autonome de la Santé (SAS), began a unique kind of strike. Continuing to provide health care to the general population, government health workers began to withhold routine patient data from the central Ministry of Health. Because the workers' strike did not cripple the health system in an immediate sense and because talks between the unions and the Senegalese government hit stalemate after stalemate, the strike persisted until March 2013. This means that from 2010 to 2013 the Senegalese Ministry of Health and its international and private partners had little or incomplete national data and the health community functioned with very limited or speculative data.

The 2010–13 health worker data retention strike was the second of its kind in Senegal. The first, lasting from 1998 until 2002, was inspired by a teachers union strike in which teachers continued their work but withheld students' grades from the Ministry of Education as a means to bring the government to the table to deal with the union's demands for better working conditions. The 2010–13 SUTSAS-SAS strike had twenty-seven explicit demands, including an increase in the number of admittances to the national public health education system (Ecole Nationale de Développement Sanitaire et Sociale), the ratification of the international Convention on the Rights of Persons with Disabilities, and various demands on increasing pay for hospital workers. The demand for better working conditions was largely geared toward urban health workers, as they would benefit those with more training. However, health workers in health huts, posts, and centers across every sector adhered to the strike, and, problematically, the rural health workers were even *more* militant about adhering to it than hospital workers and urban health workers. This was problematic because these health workers were not going to benefit from the fruits of the strike should the government address the union convergence's demands (which it largely did not) and also because this meant that there was relatively complete data for those health districts in urban areas and an almost complete lack of data for those districts in rural regions. Because the NMCP uses these data to construct its strategies, it broadened the gap between rural and urban health care even further and impeded its ability to deal with malaria in rural areas.

The data retention strike was also linked to the unions' desire to highlight the problem of a lack of equipment and infrastructure throughout the Senegalese health system. In this way it was part of a larger trend in sub-Saharan Africa of an increasing "willingness of the labor movement to be present in the political arena, not only with regards to worker demands—which is quite logical and consistent with its mission—but also in terms of the rights and duties of citizens beyond their status as workers" (Floridi et al. 2008: 71). The official stance of the union convergence, as explained to me in an interview, was that this kind of strike was a means "to humanize the struggle" both for better working conditions and for a "health care financially and geographically accessible to all." Because health workers continued to provide care, they argued, this form of struggling for workers rights and universal adequate health coverage allowed health workers to remain at the side of those who needed their aid while also making a political statement.

There is much disagreement within the union convergence about whether or not the strike actually humanized the struggle for better national health care. Dissenters from within called the strike "extremist" and pointed to the fact that it was the poor people of Senegal in particular who would suffer from a strike like this and that the unions should not be content to better their own means and not the country in general. One of the key issues of the dissenters was how long the strike lasted; they believed the leadership's call to strike should have been constantly and responsibly revisited.

Describing the health worker unions as the "sentinels of the health system," a representative of the convergence emphasized the fact that they supported a health system that depended on a working relationship between the government and the health workers. The government, he said, should be taking advantage of the fact that it is the health workers who can see what the real problems are and what needs to be addressed. This representative believed that the breakdown with the strike, and why it lasted so long, was due to the fact that the government refused to listen to the health workers, despite the fact that the health workers were in a unique position to give advice to the government on what works and does not work in the national health system.

Although the official union opinion did not acknowledge the role of the strike in the relationship between the government and the international community, I spoke with one union member who stated that the strike was a conscious move on the part of the two health worker unions to disrupt the relationship between the Senegalese state and the international health development partners working in Senegal. By withholding the data that external aid partners and NGOs need to justify their programs in Senegal, the striking health workers were putting the Senegalese government in a very uncomfortable position: it was fundamentally responsible for providing the evidence needed to justify aid, but it was unwilling or unable to accommodate the demands of the union convergence. This meant that the union convergence and the Senegalese government held the other accountable for the damage being wrought by a lack of data and that the lack of data itself was disrupting the Senegalese state's partnerships that were so crucial to the success of health campaigns in the country.[4]

The NMCP and its international and private partners viewed the data retention strike as the largest roadblock to the adequate provision of care on a countrywide level and as creating a problem that would haunt the health sector for years to come. The strike lingered even as the global health apparatus demanded more thorough data monitoring and evaluation and as new "data management tools" continued to be rolled out, requiring new forms of training for all health workers. Many public health workers in Dakar expressed frustration that any training they would do in rural regions would be useless because, they suspected, most health workers were not only withholding data from the Ministry of Health but were simply not collecting data at all. Despite the fact that part of the effort by health workers was to complicate the relationship of Senegal with its international donors, the donor community's view of the situation was much less nuanced. According to one representative of the international aid community in Dakar, the strike showed a "lack of maturity" on the part of the union members: "They do not understand the impacts of their own actions, and the only reason the strike ended was because of the fact that the minister of health used to be a member of one of the unions."

As we can see, understandings of the rationale behind this strike vary widely within the health world in Senegal. However, it is universally acknowledged that the damage the strike has inflicted on the health system in the long term is great, that the specific long-term effects are largely unknown, and that the work of reestablishing exhaustive, regular reporting practices and of recouping the missing data from 2010 to 2013 has been and will be vast. Keeping this in mind, I argue that the health data retention strike is a novel form of political resistance that is articulated particularly within the paradigm of health governance as it currently exists in Senegal.

As the strike pushed against the current network of state and nonstate, national and international entities that control the centrally distributed funds for the public health system in Senegal—a system that is highly dependent on the kind of information that doctors and nurses gather about their patients—it also served as a critique of what is frequently overlooked by health policymakers. In order to monitor current health initiatives and projects and to design and implement new ones, particularly with regard to the local fights against HIV/AIDS, tuberculosis, malaria, and malnutrition, the Senegalese Ministry of Health and its international donors depend heavily on data received nationwide about diagnoses, prescribed treatment regimens, and pharmaceutical side effects (pharmacovigilance). Before the *mot d'ordre* was issued by SUTSAS and SAS in July 2010 these data were supposed to be recorded at public health facilities and reported to the central medical establishment once every month.

The data retention strike makes clear how critical aspects of a functioning health system are routinely overlooked in countries that receive aid to combat malaria. A critically functioning health system today includes a sufficient number and distribution of trained health workers, supply infrastructure that works most of the time, and properly stocked and available health posts, centers, or hospitals for rural populations. The lack of human resources in Senegal is often described as a barrier to health that needs to be overcome through the vigilance of donor organizations. Donor organizations in turn (and USAID in particular) assert that they can provide only consulting on human resources policies that the Senegalese government has designed.

In the case of the data retention strike, the international community did not interfere in the talks between the government and the unions, and it resisted intervening in problems that donors felt were the responsibility of the Senegalese government and its management of health workers. However, the strike eventually ended in part due to pressure from the international community. In particular, negative media presentations of the strike and the damage it was doing to the country's ability to reach the Millennium Development Goals were used to exert pressure on the strikers. In the press during the last months of the strike there was an increased emphasis on campaigns that articulated the relationship between reaching the Millennium Development Goals and the strike's ability to make achieving those goals impossible, labeling the strikers "utopian" and out of touch with the realities facing the country. These campaigns talked about how the strike prevented the "evolution of health indicators" or the threat of a health system that seemed to be "navigated without a compass" (Le Secretariat du Comité Central du PIT 2011). Ultimately these appeals to health workers aimed to make them feel that they were failing to provide health care because they were failing to provide the kinds of statistical information that could be used to expand the metrics upon which governance and funding relied. We can investigate the often problematic interplay of these twin demands on individual health workers with a trip to southeast Senegal.

The National Malaria Control Program's Pharmaceutical
Evaluation and Survey Team Goes to the Field

The road from the health district center in Goudiri to the tiny rural health post of Sinthiou Mamadou is deteriorating. It's the fourth and final day of the NMCP's Pharmaceutical Evaluation and Survey team's routine supervision trip to the southeast region of Tambacounda, and both Soxna and I are exhausted from the constant travel. The first day brought us from Dakar to the Mauritanian border at the town of Bakel, which took more than twelve hours of travel. But even my tiredness and aches feel privileged: we travel in an air-conditioned 4x4. I tell her that it's odd that, despite the fact that we are doing it in such luxury, traveling is so tiring. She smiles faintly and agrees. Like me, Soxna is an intern with NMCP; she is particularly interested in the distribution of long-lasting insecticidal nets. She is about to receive her doctorate in pharmacology from the medical school at the University of Cheikh Anta Diop, and her research focuses on the use of medicinal plants at one of the largest public hospitals in Senegal. Her work with the NMCP is a necessary step for obtaining her master's degree in public health.

But the road: it's eighteen kilometers from Goudiri to Sinthiou Mamadou, and it's falling apart. It's only a dirt road, but it obviously hasn't been maintained for years. We almost get stuck because the hard-packed dirt has started to crack and crumble in the middle and falls away into ditches on either side. I think about how people get around on these roads without 4x4s and how often people have to travel this distance, how many people live even farther than Sinthiou Mamadou from Goudiri. They must have to travel that distance because there aren't any stores in these outlying villages. In order to get tea and sugar and rice and any manufactured goods, people have to travel this disintegrating road by foot or by motorcycle.

I was at first surprised by how sparsely populated this part of Senegal is compared to the eastern border towns we had been in earlier. It quickly became clear why: the Senegal River flows along the border between Senegal and Mauritania and then between Senegal and Mali, and it cuts through the Sahel and the Soudan and creates a bustling economy on both sides of the length of the borders. Development projects exist all along it, to ameliorate irrigation, to provide microloans, to empower women, and so on. But Goudiri is some forty kilometers from the Senegal River, and the dry Sahel heat is in full force here. It's unclear to me what people do to keep food in their mouths here, how they survive the summer heat (I'm already sweating in February), what they can cultivate from this dry, red sand.

When we arrive at the health post, both Soxna and I are queasy, and we stumble through the gates. They're constructing a new health post on the left-hand side, but there's still a lot of work to be done. Much of the financing for these health posts and schools in the remote rural areas of Senegal depends heavily on investment in the communities by those who have migrated to the *grandes villes* in Senegal or out of the country altogether. Needless to say, construction is slow, and it looks like the new health post has been in the midst of construction for quite some time. The working health post is on the right, and it is falling apart. There are no steps to get up to the raised platform, only a single cement block, and once again I wonder about how people less mobile than I manage with these kinds of inconveniences. How does an elderly gentleman with serious arthritis or a very pregnant woman deal with this cement block?

The *infirmière chef de poste* (ICP), the nurse and the head of the health post, comes out from her compound through a gate on the right. She is all smiles and has her adorable infant daughter strapped to her back. Soxna explains who we are, and there's some confusion. The Goudiri district *médicin chef de district* neglected to inform her that we were coming, and she is not prepared for us. We apologize profusely, but she's not worried and leads us to her main office, the first room of the crumbling building. She explains that she is the only permanent staff at the health post, performing the role of ICP, *sage femme* (midwife), pharmacist, and anything else that might come up. Soxna looks up in alarm, then turns to me and says, "You understand that, right? She has no pharmacist. She is the only one working here. Make sure you write that down." I nod furiously and scratch it all down in my notebook.

Our role here is now ridiculous: our main goal with this supervision trip is to go to a handful of posts, whatever we can hit in three days over massive distances in the region of Tambacounda, and assess the conditions of the drug depots and the training levels of the local pharmacists. This is part of an effort to make widespread specific "rational" practices of drug management, including methods of reporting and stocking, which is how the official documentation of the trip has defined this work. In an effort to rationalize the distribution of pharmaceuticals, we have been sent out to southern regions to figure out the problems and to consider possible solutions. The southern regions are where malaria is the biggest problem (partly because of transmission rates and the fact that the rainy season lasts longer there than anywhere else in the country) and where health infrastructure is the weakest. What is really lacking at the health post of Sinthiou Mamadou, however, is *other health workers*. And yet the only time of the year that the ICP seems to need this extra help is during the rainy season, when the transmission rate for malaria is highest and when she has to personally treat more than 150 patients a month. During the rest of the year she normally treats around twenty-five to thirty-five patients a month.

There was a pharmacist here when this ICP first arrived, but he left a couple months after she started work. However, as the ICP told us, it is difficult to find replacements for these kinds of positions because "les enfants ici n'apprennent pas": the children here do not learn. Most of the students make it through only a couple years of school and do not master French writing and speaking. The connection between educational opportunities and the disappearing pharmacist was not clear until a few hours later, when, near the end of our supervision of the health post in Sinthiou Mamadou, I went out to the car to pick up the packet of "data management tools" we brought with us to give to the ICP. This was a monthly reporting book on specific medicines prescribed and given, a record of stocked medicines, and a book full of ordering sheets that would get sent to the health district pharmaceutical depot in Goudiri to be filled. Right next to the health post was the local school, and a crowd of children of varying ages was sitting in front on a break. As I walked to where Sidy, our driver, had parked the car under one of the few nearby trees, the crowd came ambling toward me. This was a common experience in rural Senegal: the color of my skin marked me with undeserved celebrity. All of the children began to shout at me, "Bonjour, Madame! Comment ça va?!" My arms full of data management tools, I couldn't shake their hands, which is common practice, and so I tried to say "Bonjour! Ça va?" in response to each child. I wondered how the ICP must have felt surrounded by the youthful aspirations of children like this, knowing the obstacles that lie in their path to becoming the kind of workers who would or could return to the area to work.

On our way back to Goudiri, Soxna tells me that this is a common occurrence in this area of Senegal. In the sparsely populated regions it is hard to find educated workers who want to stay in the area rather than go where work opportunities are better. Few of these students will ever be able to do health work, even though they might be the most likely to want to return. And so these rural health posts have limited staff, and people come from great distances to be treated at a poorly stocked and staffed health post. As a result the ICP is often the only person to take care of all the health services and all of the surveillance and data collection and management tasks that rural clinics like this are asked to fulfill. It is simply too much for one person. That the system requires local health workers to take on these enormous responsibilities while simultaneously taking the brunt of the logistical obstacles intrinsic within that system is not new (see Justice 1986), and there is no known solution for this kind of problem.[5]

Under these conditions the correct reporting of how many treatments of antimalarials the ICP has received from the district depot is not her priority. In fact her way of dealing with what Steven Feierman (2010) has called the "normal emergency" of often insufficient health care in rural Senegal flies directly in the face of her duty to record things precisely: she is invested in stocking up as much as possible for the high malarial transmission season. In her case, reporting on how many treatments she has stored in her pharmaceutical cabinet—shelves stuffed full of different forms of Winthrop ACTs (for infants, children, and adults)—would have raised eyebrows at the district level, but this was her way of protecting her patients from the inevitable stock outs that plague the public health system. Her way of navigating a faulty distribution system was in direct contradiction to the "rationalization" of practices that the NMCP was so keen to enforce. And yet Soxna's reluctance to report on the ICP's improvisational methods in our summary of the trip shows how data production in the field is always a creative process, even by those sent to enforce "rational" practices.

Data Management and Everything Else

In her ethnography of AIDS researchers in Malawi, Crystal Biruk (2012) shows how volunteers who gather data about disease incidence and cases use and complicate categories, identities, and practices through the act of quantification. The numbers produced in these contexts are assumed to be representative of the everyday realities with which these volunteers come into contact, and the numbers are taken as a whole to abstract the idea of "Malawi" and the country's incidence of AIDS in an international context. The data production of public health workers in Senegal similarly exemplifies how the recording of numbers—assumed, or maybe hoped, to be neutral by international funding agencies—is always already a sociocultural process.

At Sinthiou Mamadou the NMCP must confront and contend with the sheer lack of human and material resources. As the NMCP pharmaceutical monitoring team went into the field, we could see with our own eyes the collision of purposes that was built into the multipronged approach to providing "rational" health care to the Senegalese population. The NMCP received designated funds from USAID-PMI for this trip and the many like it that took place in the winter of 2012 and the spring of 2013 throughout Senegal's seventy-four health districts. This antimalarial-focused drug monitoring system was set up and supported by the Global Fund during the fourth and seventh rounds of funding. However, the Global Fund stopped funding "this important program for improving the management of antimalarial commodities in peripheral health structures" in 2010 (NMCP 2013a), and USAID-PMI stepped in to fill the funding gap, as has been commonplace in the past decade of the fight against malaria in Senegal.[6]

The data production on the ordering and use of antimalarials that the NMCP team evaluated in 2012–13 in "peripheral structures" in the regions outside of urban areas is only a small part of the large body of data that health workers are required to generate as part of their quotidian activities. The programs within the Ministry of Health are quite fragmented; each has its own budget and its own objectives focused on a single disease or condition, like malaria, malnutrition, or tuberculosis. These programs are nested in *directions* or departments of the Ministry of Health, and each has its own demands on the data-producing labor of health workers. The programs themselves are at the mercy of the funding or intervening international organizations that ask for accountability, and the kinds of data these organizations ask for often change. According to one member of SUTSAS, the "health directions are too demanding—they are constantly changing protocols and someone is always calling for a summary of data that may or may not already exist." This union member was particularly frustrated with the demands the NMCP was making with regard to recouping the malarial data over the period of the 2010–13 data retention strike.

The NMCP needs to secure data on how its initiatives are working and will work in the future, and the Global Fund demands that the program recoup data that health workers were thought to have been recording throughout the period of the strike. Thus the data that health workers collect is not tied tightly to the act of providing care—routine patient data are not a reflection or easy representation of what actually happens in consultation rooms or microscopy laboratories in health structures. Instead, these data take on many different meanings and do many kinds of work. Providing data from the three-year period of the strike required many workers to create data entirely, as many actually had not been collecting data or the right kind of data during that time. Workers produced an image of the general trends they were seeing, working with the sparse records they did have to flesh out the edges. They were attempting to create an acceptable reality for those to whom they were accountable. As many other authors in this volume argue, pre-inscribed health indicators limit the kinds of data and the kinds of questions that can be asked about the health of populations at large. This sometimes wholesale production of health data, with respect to existing health indicators, in the wake of the data retention strike makes clear the disconnection of the experience of illness and health in places like Senegal and the evidence that governors of global health require from countries for participation.

The Power of Locally Produced Health Data: Responsibilities of a Global Health Citizen

The data retention strike indeed took a toll on the security of the country's funding of malaria interventions from the Global Fund in 2013. Because the Senegalese NMCP was unable to provide data from across the country, the Global Fund put Senegal on the list of countries that were not eligible for grant applications for their malaria programs in mid-2013. The program and its partners were able to convince the Fund that the strike had finally ended in March 2013 and that they needed six more months to work on collecting, analyzing, and synthesizing the data. When I left they were in the process of review.

In its assessment of Senegal's use of funds for the fight against malaria (last updated in August 2013), the Global Fund had this to say:

> The poor performance of [Senegal's NMCP] grant is mainly linked to the lack of availability of data to appropriately report on output indicators in the performance framework. The lack of available data is not under the control of the [NMCP] or other partners, but is related to the strike of health care workers who have retained data transmission to the district and central level in protest of poor salaries since 2010. The strikes ended in March 2013. It is to be noted that a retrospective collection of data from the health centers is being conducted by both

[NMCP] and [the National Health Information System]. The goal of this exercise is the recuperation of existing data since the start of the program." (Global Fund 2013)[7]

When I left Senegal in August 2013, the collection of data had still not been completed, although the heads of the medical districts were working hard to recover data from all levels within their health districts and there was the expectation that the NMCP would be more efficient at recouping the data on their own, rather than with the National Health Information System, and would be able to provide the Global Fund the data by the deadline the funding agency had given them. During the drawn out process to recoup data, which was still continuing upon my return to Senegal in the spring of 2014, Senegal's NMCP received a two year grant from the Global Fund, to fund activities from January 2015 to December 2017. Thus, though the strike and the tension it created produced a rupture to view the political relations between health workers and the international donor community, the problems that the strikers brought up were easily smoothed over in the name of maintaining the local industry around the health fight against malaria.

We can see how notions of accountability and citizenship in Senegal are caught up in the production of health data because of current global health governance's framing concept of performance-based funding and its focus on metrics as justifying evidence. With their demands and the way they chose to strike, the SUTSAS-SAS convergence members highlighted that the practices of accountability that each level requires of health workers in the public sector (the health district, the Ministry of Health, the Senegalese state, the state's external partners, and the international organizations that govern them) are dissociated from and at times overshadow the actual provision of health care. Through this strike health workers also showed that these practices constitute what it means to be a proper global health citizen. A health worker's labor as data producer is essential to her country's admittance to that global system of governance as well as, through her national citizenship, her own individual admittance.

Taking the case of the Senegalese data retention strike along with the more visible case of the data retention strike of 2007 in Indonesia, we can see how local health data, in the always already interconnected relationships of global health, produce value in many ways and complicate the questions of ownership over local action. These two cases also show how the valuation of locally produced health data is a process that has stakes

l health governance. The production of health data today perpetu-
equal power relations between the Global North and the Global
. Like Susan Erikson's (2012) example of "data performativity" in
ductive health in Sierra Leone and Germany, Senegal's data retention strike highlights the ways that global health must be enumerated in
order to work. In the Indonesian case, the government's refusal to produce
data for the WHO's Global Influenza Surveillance Network was presented
by some in the international media as a moral failing and as "irrational"
(Lakoff 2010), as hindering the international community's ability to combat a potential pandemic. However, Indonesia's refusal also pointed to the
very important fact that its participation in the global health system far
from guaranteed its ability to protect its own citizenry from a pandemic, a
fact that was not always presented by the media.

The 2010–13 Senegalese health data retention strike shows how, even
within a regime of humanitarian biomedicine, countries and their workers
have the ability to engage with the requirements for data production that
serve global health efforts in unique and not always predictable ways. Participation in these regimes of data production does not necessarily guarantee the provision of health care to a country's own citizenry or the provision
of social security to those who produce the data and provide services, but
participation in these data regimes and accepting global health governance
are requirements for access to global health markets. The problems that the
SUTSAS-SAS convergence raised with regard to the distribution of health resources and accessibility to sustainable employment within Senegal deserve
attention. The ease with which the media discounted the strike and the fact
that the strike did not succeed in achieving its demands unfortunately also
point to the massive obstacles that stand in the way of achieving health globally in a "more democratic and equitable manner" (Geissler 2011: 2).

The infrastructural and personnel shortages that plague the health system in Senegal, so visible at a health post like Sinthiou Mamadou's, are
invisible to a global health assemblage that defines success by the slow advancement toward the elimination of malaria. The disruption of reporting
on Senegal's level of success in this goal is a novel form of political resistance that appeals to both a national and a global sovereign. However, the
ease with which the strike was overlooked shows that the production of
health data at times eclipses the provision of care and that such productivity is integral to not only health but also to national governance in places
like Senegal.

Notes

1. The Roll Back Malaria Partnership (2010) reports that investment in malaria R&D increased from $121 million in 1993 to $612 million in 2009, and the Bill and Melinda Gates Foundation (2014b) reports that R&D quadrupled again to an estimated $2 billion in 2011. PATH (2010) reports that "between 2004 and 2009, 38% of R&D funds were invested in drugs, 28% in vaccines, 23% in basic research, 4% in vector control products and 1% in diagnostics."

2. In 2007 experts worried that a global influenza pandemic was inevitable if a particularly virulent strain of the H5N1 virus (which infected birds) was able to mutate and infect humans. Most cases of this strain of H5N1 were occurring in Indonesia, but the government refused to share its samples of the virus with the WHO's Global Influenza Surveillance Network, which had been set up in the 1950s as an "early warning system" to prepare for a major outbreak on a global scale. The root reason for its withholding of biological data was that the Indonesian government had discovered that an Australian pharmaceutical company had begun developing a vaccine with the H5N1 strain. Their worry was that this company would develop a vaccine that would be unaffordable and inaccessible for the Indonesian population itself.

3. The Bamako Initiative, sponsored by the WHO and UNICEF, was a statement accepted by African heads of state in 1987 in response to the reality that, particularly in sub-Saharan Africa, many countries receiving international development aid continued to lack the resources to meet the goals of increasing quality and access to primary health care (which was itself a goal accepted by heads of state with the Declaration of Alma Ata in 1978). The Bamako Initiative aimed to increase access to suitable health care for populations at large by focusing on access to drugs and increased contact between communities at large and the health care workers who serve them. It attempted to increase the effectiveness of health care, defined by these two goals, by leveraging user fees and drug costs from those who seek health care, thereby creating a local fund to support the running of community health centers (United Nations Children's Rights and Emergency Relief Organization 2007).

4. This perspective can be seen in the commentary of the Senegalese newspaper Le Soleil on the resolution of the strike in March 2013: "Mais en fait, quel est l'impact de l'information sanitaire sur le système? L'inexistence de données est un obstacle à l'élaboration de toutes les stratégies de lutte contre les maladies. Au-delà, la rétention a des incidences négatives sur le partenariat. 'Si vous n'avez pas de données, vous ne pouvez bâtir une stratégie pertinente en matière de lutte. Le bulletin épidémiologique sénégalais n'existe pas au plan international,' a souligné le syndicaliste Mballo Dia Thiam." "But what indeed is the impact of health data on the health system? The lack of data is an obstacle to the elaboration of all of the strategies for fighting diseases. Beyond that, the retention has negative effects on partnership. 'If you don't have the data, you cannot create an effective strategy in the fight. The Senegalese epidemiological bulletin does not exist internationally,' emphasizes unionist Mballo Dia Thiam" (Sane 2013).

5. In recent years the Senegalese Ministry of Health and its funding partners have made the lack of human resources a central issue in the improvement of public health care. It is included within the 2009–18 National Plan for Health Development as a

problem to address (Ministry of Health and Prevention of Senegal 2009). Additionally SUTSAS has identified it as a key obstacle to their goal of universal health coverage (Thiam 2013). The impacts of this increased attention to the labor problem are yet to be seen.

6. The highly bureaucratic nature of the Global Fund was a constant source of frustration for NMCP and its public and private partners. There is often a large lag between the promise of money and its actual delivery, which disrupts the very schedule of project development that the Global Fund itself requires for continued funding, with regard to its performance-based funding principles.

7. It is important to note the exceptionality of the health fight against malaria in Senegal. While the NMCP was greatly dependent on the data movement chains that existed within the Senegalese health system, the National Council against AIDS was not. The funding for the local fight against HIV/AIDS was not at stake in the same way that the funding for malaria was due to the data retention strike.

5 · NATIVE SOVEREIGNTY BY THE NUMBERS

The Metrics of Yup'ik Behavioral Health Programs   MOLLY HALES

On a warm July afternoon I sat in a conference room in Tundra Flats, Alaska, where a coalition of about fifteen representatives from the town's various social service agencies were gathered to share updates and plan joint projects.[1] I was doing preliminary fieldwork with Tundra Flats's public health nursing program and had accompanied the nurse manager to the meeting.[2] Sally, a middle-aged Yup'ik woman from the native health corporation's Behavioral Health Department, was describing a new program that was being introduced into the villages, Principles of Health. Someone handed me a brochure:

> The Tundra Flats Regional Health Corporation through its newly established Preventative Services Department implements and disseminates the traditional and community-based program, [Principles of Health] in our communities throughout the . . . region in partnership with regional, tribal and local organizations.

The Yup'ik-based curriculum builds upon traditional and pre-scribed ways-of-living. These values orally passed down by the wisdom of our Yup'ik Elders are then developed into a curriculum that aims to address families and communities to building and strengthening family units utilizing these traditions.

Sally explained that the three-day Principles of Health training would reintroduce participants to the wisdom that had long guided Yupiit (plural of Yup'ik) through difficult times. She and her colleagues had recently offered the training in several nearby villages and had met a warm reception. Several representatives from other organizations chimed in that they'd heard of the great success of Principles of Health.

As Sally wrapped up, someone spoke up from the end of the table: "The challenge now is to figure out how to measure it!"

Evidence-based practices are reshaping behavioral health programs in rural Alaska.[3] As state and private funders demand new forms of statistical accountability, native agencies must scramble to capture the efficacy of their health programs without compromising their own core values in the process.

The work in this volume joins recent literature in drawing attention to the ways that global formations—including global health institutions and structures—can supersede and cross-cut nation-states (Adams, chapter 1, this volume; Bartelson 2006; Comaroff and Comaroff 2001; Hardt and Negri 2001; Howland and White 2009; Ong 2006). Such insights are significant to native and nonnative communities alike. Yet it is important to locate the emergence of this new global sovereign within existing struggles over the sovereign status of indigenous peoples living in ongoing conditions of colonialism.[4] Many indigenous groups continue to fight for the rights associated with classic definitions of sovereignty: rights to a bounded territory, control over resources and their distribution, political recognition from other states, and autonomous governance of their citizens (Cattelino 2008; Deloria and Lytle 1984; Howland and White 2009; Huhndorf and Huhndorf 2011; Kalt et al. 2007; McCarrey 2013; Wilkinson 2005).[5] For such peoples, including many Yupiit, sovereignty is critically important to protecting livelihood and preserving a sense of authenticity. In what follows I use the term *post/colonial* to underscore the extent to which indigenous peoples such as the Yupiit continue to exist under conditions of colonial occupation, even as they have entered into the "architectures of debt and finance" that have marked the shift from colonial to postcolonial.[6]

In the unfolding global health landscape of the twenty-first century, the legitimacy conferred by health metrics plays a complicated role in struggles for indigenous sovereignty. By making funding for Yup'ik behavioral health programs contingent on the production of health metrics, the post/colonial settler-state perpetuates relationships of financial and intellectual dependency. This is one way global health aspirations towards a contemporary "global sovereign" dovetail with long-standing colonial histories to ensure the perpetuation of colonial dependencies in indigenous communities (Adams, chapter 1, this volume). Yet metrics can also be mobilized by indigenous communities themselves. Even as they dispute the purported universality of health metrics, the directors of Yup'ik behavioral health search for creative ways to demonstrate evidence of efficacy. They are cognizant of the ways health metrics confer legitimacy to an international audience and may help instantiate their claims to sovereignty.

Before moving to a more detailed consideration of the relationship between global health metrics and Yup'ik sovereignty, it is necessary to briefly review the recent history of Alaska Native sovereignty struggles, as well as the current politico-economic status of Alaska Native groups.

Tribal Sovereignty and Corporate Governance

In 1971 President Richard Nixon signed into law the Alaska Native Claims Settlement Act (ANCSA), addressing long-standing native land claims that had been deferred since the acquisition of the Territory of Alaska from Russia in 1867. Defying precedents set by U.S. dealings with Native American tribes, ANCSA did not grant land rights and financial compensation to tribes.[7] Instead, Congress created thirteen for-profit regional corporations and 225 village corporations,[8] which were granted rights to land and funds under existing Alaska corporate law (Linxwiler 2007:49). Alaska Natives who were born before 1971 were enrolled as "shareholders" in regional corporations, and those residing in rural Alaska at the time were simultaneously enrolled in village corporations (Huhndorf and Huhndorf 2011).[9] Shareholders were issued one hundred shares of corporate stock, making them eligible to receive distributions of corporate revenues (McCarrey 2013: 445).

ANCSA was an experiment in assimilationist policy. With it, Congress converted land that was collectively used by native people into allotments of private property owned by corporations. Although it was native *groups* that were seeking financial compensation, the funds that were awarded were incorporated into a system of corporate dividends to be distributed to *individual* native shareholders. The original ANCSA provisions also allowed native shareholders to sell their corporate stock after twenty years, bringing native lands and restitution funds into the free market.[10] ANCSA was thus intended to introduce Alaska Natives into the market economy, to instantiate a self-interested individualism among native people, and to eventually erode the territorial and economic basis of shared native identity.

Furthermore, ANCSA failed to elaborate on the sovereign status of Alaska Natives, avoiding the issue of political recognition. In the lower forty-eight states, relationships between Native American governments and federal and state governments are largely based on treaties that confer "recognition" to tribes.[11] Recognized Native American tribes are political bodies with jurisdiction over a bounded territory (reservations), the right to establish qualifications for citizenship (such as blood quanta), and basic rights of self-government, such as the ability to establish independent educational, health, and legal systems using funding from contracts and compacts with the Bureau of Indian Affairs (Kalt et al. 2007; Wilkinson 2005).[12] These rights and recognitions are often collectively referred to as "tribal sovereignty" or "native sovereignty" by legal experts, scholars in Native American studies, and native people themselves.

The treaties that conferred tribal sovereignty to Native Americans resulted from violent clashes during U.S. expansion in the eighteenth and nineteenth centuries. By escaping overt attack, Alaska Natives were ironically denied the opportunity to sign treaties with the federal government. In subsequent years Alaska Natives have fought to achieve legal recognition of their sovereign status through numerous court battles, with inconsistent results. A 1996 court decision found that ANCSA villages counted as "tribes," provided that they could trace their origin to a "historic tribe." However, a subsequent U.S. Supreme Court decision found that these tribes did *not* have territorial jurisdiction over ANCSA corporate land, raising questions about the meaning of sovereignty in the absence of a land base governed by a recognized tribal government (Huhndorf and Huhndorf 2011).

Although Alaska Native governments do not have jurisdiction over native land, they do have a degree of control over health and social services. Through contracts and compacts, funds that have been earmarked for Alaska Natives can be transferred from the federal Bureau of Indian Affairs to the native institutions of governance. These native institutions can then directly provide services such as education, housing, and health care and can determine the scope and content of these programs (Kalt et al. 2007). Anthropologist Jessica Cattelino (2008) refers to such forms of tribal administration as sites of "sovereignty-in-the making," blurring the distinction between sovereignty and governmentality.[13]

For Yupiit, behavioral health programs are particularly rich sites of native sovereignty-in-the-making. Yup'ik behavioral health programs set local knowledge alongside medical expertise in order to address the range of difficulties that Yup'ik families face in the wake of a century and a half of disruptive post/colonial management by the U.S. government and the state of Alaska.[14] The content of behavioral health programs and the manner in which they are funded take on added significance as enactments of native sovereignty and challenges to post/colonialism.

Sovereignty and Dependency: The Dilemma of Funding Yup'ik Behavioral Health Programs

In 2008 the tribal government of Tundra Flats began offering a parenting class based on local knowledge gathered from Yup'ik elders' oral histories. The curriculum is organized around a "cycle of life" model that was originally proposed by a respected elder and community leader, and then subsequently refined in a gathering of elders in 2010. According to the organizational literature, the cycle of life incorporates Yup'ik *nutemllaat*, or principles, that have long assured the health and wellness of Yupiit.[15] The original parenting class has since been joined by several related programs: Healing Our Relationships, which is also run by the local tribal government; Healing Our Families, which is run by the regional native nonprofit; and Principles of Health, which is offered by the native health corporation. While the institutional support and target audience of these programs vary, each proposes to reeducate Yup'ik participants in the lifeways of their ancestors as a means of addressing issues such as alcohol use, interpartner violence, child abuse and neglect, and suicide. The persistence of these problems has long been used to justify intervention from outside experts in the medical and public health fields, backed by federal and state governments (Jones 2004; Stevenson 2012). Such interventions perpetuate long-standing colonial dependencies while simultaneously framing these dependencies in a post/colonial language of "help" and "assistance" to the needy. (See Stevenson 2014 for an insightful analysis of a similar dynamic between the Canadian settler-state and the Inuit.) By offering programs such as Healing Our Families and Principles of Health, Yupiit push against these post/colonial power dynamics. They assert that they are capable of healing their own people.

The *content* of Yup'ik behavioral health programs further challenge U.S. post/colonial practices. Collectively their curricula suggest that colonialism itself is to blame for behavioral health struggles. During a conversation about Principles of Health, one of the program organizers told me, "The people in our region, before subjugation, they were *thriving*. And for how long? Millennia! Twenty-five thousand to forty thousand years." Program leaders emphasize that colonization threatened native livelihoods, disrupted local structures of communal assistance and eroded the knowledge base that allowed Yupiit to effectively address emotional challenges. Yup'ik behavioral health programs link the devastation caused by colonialism to ongoing experiences of emotional distress. For example, the three-day Principles of Health workshop begins with a day-long exploration of "historical trauma," a concept developed in the 1980s to illustrate the ways that trauma can be passed from generation to generation.[16] Sally, one of the directors, reported that Principles of Health participants have been "awed" by these colonial histories and that the concept of historical trauma provides an opening in which "stories come out."

Thus Yup'ik behavioral health programs affirm native sovereignty and challenge post/colonial framings of native struggles. Their curricula reverse existing lines of causation, shifting responsibility for Yup'ik suffering from native people themselves to the state and federal governments and assistance programs that claim to be acting out of concern for Yup'ik well-being. Unfortunately, assimilationist federal policies ensure that these behavioral health programs remain financially dependent on state and federal funding, reintroducing post/colonial power dynamics into instances of indigenous self-governance.

ANCSA purported to offer an alternative form of autonomy to native peoples, based not on tribal jurisdiction over reservations and their residents but on *economic* advancement secured through the pursuit of corporate profit (Huhndorf and Huhndorf 2011: 386). But by tying revenues to a corporate structure that is obligated by law to prioritize the generation of profits for individual shareholders, ANCSA left native governments and social service agencies bereft of funding and dependent on the goodwill of state, federal, and private granting agencies (Kalt et al. 2007). In other words, because ANCSA is structured on a model of *individual* financial profit, the regional native corporations are not equipped to provide significant financial support to native institutions of governance, such as health and social service agencies.

As a result, Yup'ik behavioral health programs face significant budgetary constraints. Their structures of debt and finance exist at the intersection of colonial and postcolonial dependencies. Although the state of Alaska and the U.S. federal government continue to fund much of the region's health care—including Tundra Flats's behavioral health programs—they do so increasingly through short-term grants that mimic the private-sector funding provided by NGOs and humanitarian agencies in many global health settings (Adams chapter 1, Erikson, and Walkover, all this volume).

Principles of Health is administered by the Behavioral Health Department of the regional native health corporation, which also runs the regional hospital as well as a collection of village clinics.[17] Faced with budget shortfalls in the range of nearly $12 million, the health corporation has recently had to lay off nearly 10 percent of its staff. Native health care leaders have been actively seeking to increase funding from third-party providers, as well as from public and private grants, to meet the shortfall. Grant funding is a particularly significant portion of the budget of the Behavioral Health Department, which received approximately $4.6 million in grant revenue in 2013.

The Healing Our Families program faces even greater financial uncertainty. Healing Our Families is run by the regional native nonprofit, a consortium of native villages that pool the funding they receive from the Bureau of Indian Affairs to administer public services. Bureau of Indian Affairs funding is notoriously scant, compelling the regional native nonprofit to compete for additional funding from state, federal, and private sources. For its first few years Healing Our Families was funded by a three-year grant from the state of Alaska. In my first year in Tundra Flats this grant period was drawing to a close, and program directors were attempting to gather evidence that they hoped would support their grant renewal application.

The financial dependencies that Yup'ik behavioral health programs face undermine native autonomy and contradict the federal government's stated goal of self-determination for Native American tribes (Kalt 2007: 20–21).[18] The fact that Yup'ik agencies "voluntarily" apply for grants thinly masks the continuing demands placed upon them by state and federal governments. These governments continue to set priorities for native communities and to shape the form and content of their programs. Only now they do so through the expectations and stipulations laid out in the grants that *fund* these programs. These funding mechanisms breathe new life into old inequalities, introducing new techniques of post/colonial management into entrenched colonial dependencies. As a result the very site in which self-governance is enacted — Yup'ik behavioral health programs — becomes a site in which sovereignty may be compromised.

Missing the Point: The Metrics of Behavioral Health

What happens when funding for Yup'ik behavioral health programs is made contingent on particular kinds of quantifiable evidence demonstrating "efficacy"? In the previous section I tried to show that behavioral health programs' reliance on federal, state, and private grants introduces post/colonial dependencies that undermine Yup'ik sovereignty. But it is not just the *existence* of these financial dependencies that is problematic. According to some of the Yup'ik program leaders I spoke with, demands for *health metrics* may be particularly erosive to native sovereignty.

Linda is one of the leaders of the native nonprofit that runs Healing Our Families. During one of our conversations she told me about preparing the program's grant renewal application:

> I was just meeting with one of our contractors who's trying to help us evaluate our Healing Our Families program. This is the third year of our grant that funds Healing Our Families in the way that it's offered now, where we bring in people once a month. Most of it pays for just the travel, for people to come in and attend for a week. Or for three and a half days. . . .
>
> Even me, having a college degree, trying to figure out how to translate that into a grant report for the state — and what information to really collect, that would translate to something the state would understand and see as meeting certain objectives or changes in health and behavior. It's hard.

Linda underscored the foreign nature of the audit process by construing it as a form of *translation* in which the program was rendered into "something the state would understand." She told me that her college degree was an asset not because of the technical knowledge that it proffered but because her pursuit of higher education had helped acculturate her into an alternative knowledge system. This acculturation gave her an advantage in understanding the kinds of evidence that the state funding agency would consider "legitimate."

Linda went on to suggest that the forms of evidence that her nonprofit is expected to produce do not capture the value of Healing Our Families. Describing the responses of the state officials who oversee their grants, she told me:

> They still try to fit this Healing Our Families in their understanding of how to change human behavior for *their* population. And it's still expecting something different than we're expecting.
>
> When they bring that up it feels almost like a burden that's put back on us. [They say,] "Well you're not offering aftercare, so how do these families actually heal after they've come to Healing Our Families?" And then our answer is "Well, they come back! And they come back again, or they refer other family members to it." And trying to explain that we don't need that structure that they're expecting from a treatment model—it doesn't need to be structured that way. It's a lot more organic.

Linda recognized that Healing Our Families was being measured against a model of medical treatment that the program's auditors felt was universal—a standard for measuring that could be used in any place, in any culture. She, on the other hand, felt that such measures might be misleading, or worse, they might miss the point of treatment efforts altogether. "Healing," as she put it, "doesn't need to be structured that way." Again using the rubric of "us-them," she noted that "what works for *their* population" wasn't necessarily relevant for Yup'ik people.

Linda went on to dispute the auditors' very understanding of success. Referring specifically to Healing Our Families participants who struggle with alcohol use, she said, "Maybe they don't stop drinking right away, but how many people stop drinking right away after inpatient treatment? How successful are those programs?" Linda pointed out that the program auditors were concerned with capturing the effects of treatment by following up with participants and measuring behavior change. But for her, success was not contingent on long-term adherence. When I asked Linda how she would evaluate the success of Healing Our Families, she told me, "People that want to come back, or would recommend it to their friends and family, or who want to bring it to their community. And just through those three examples, I would see it as a success." In other words, the fact that participants returned to the program on their own accord demonstrated that they are getting something out of the program. According to Linda's logic, it was the *process* of healing that was significant, not necessarily the results. In fact she explicitly stated that success was not contingent on the abandonment of detrimental health practices such as excessive alcohol use. Cultural continuity, community revitalization, and family support were at least as important—and far less amenable to quantification.

In sum, broad trends toward the use of metrics in global health practices have found their way to rural Alaska, where behavioral health programs are being asked to incorporate practices of audit and accountability. Program directors such as Linda are sometimes reluctant to embrace these techniques, seeing them as part of an external system of evaluation tied to a notion of success that's inappropriate for Yupiit. In this case demands for specific kinds of accountability become a point of rupture in the dreams of sovereignty.

Yet the use of quantifiable evidence by Yup'ik behavioral health programs is far from straightforward. Even as program leaders decry the financial dependencies that drive the production of health metrics, many are interested in exploring the possibilities that metrics may hold in their ongoing struggle for Yup'ik sovereignty. In what follows, I consider the way that health metrics participate in one particular site of struggle for Yup'ik sovereignty: child welfare.

Child Welfare: Registers of Recognition

The removal of native children from their homes has been one of the most important issues of the tribal sovereignty movement. Beginning at the turn of the twentieth century, large numbers of Native American children were sent to off-reservation boarding schools as part of a new policy of "assimilation" aimed at the destruction of native polities and the erasure of native cultures (Jacobs 2011; Piatote 2013). By the second half of the twentieth century, boarding school attendance had declined, to be replaced with the large-scale removal of native children by social workers based on allegations of abuse and neglect. Between 1941 and 1978 an estimated 68 percent of native children were placed in orphanages or with white families (Kalt et al. 2007: 237). Native American activists rallied against these removals, provoking a series of congressional hearings that culminated in the passage of the Indian Child Welfare Act (Frichner 2010). The Act remains one of the most significant recognitions of tribal sovereignty, stipulating that native children who are removed from custody must be preferentially placed (in order of preference) with extended family, with other tribal members, or with native families (Kalt et al. 2007: 244–45).

Although the Indian Child Welfare Act was an important step forward, federal and state governments retain a significant degree of control over the welfare of native children. The state of Alaska's Office of Children's Services has the right to remove Yup'ik children from their homes, as well as to determine the treatment protocol that caregivers must follow to regain custody. Many Yupiit are eager to acquire control over these cases, replacing state oversight with their own methods of healing that resonate with local understandings of what a thriving family consists of. Linda reported with pride that her nonprofit had recently persuaded the Office of Children's Services to institute a new requirement stipulating that all upper-level administrators must attend a session of Healing Our Families. She saw this as a victory that allowed the native community to have a say in "who gets to work with our families." Linda hoped that attending the program would favorably influence the administrators' "beliefs and attitudes towards Healing Our Families." She reported that the Office of Children's Services administration viewed Healing Our Families as "a good thing, but not at the level of treatment."

This is where metrics become particularly significant. The representatives from the Office of Children's Services were willing to acknowledge the benefits of the Healing Our Families program for general well-being, but they were not able to see it as a form of "treatment" because it did not meet their expectations of what constituted treatment in their system. In light of this, Linda and her colleagues' efforts to collect data according to "*their* system of evaluation" may in part be motivated by the need to convince state authorities of the rigor of their program. Linda and her colleagues must play by the rules of scientific data collection to achieve the *recognition* upon which sovereignty is premised.

This is a point that requires some elaboration. I use the term *recognition* here to move between — and draw together — multiple forms of acknowledgment. Linda was specifically seeking recognition from the Office of Children's Services as to the legitimacy of Healing Our Families. But she and her colleagues' larger goal was to achieve *recognition* that the Yup'ik leadership is capable of managing the welfare of native children, without outside interventions from the state of Alaska. At present Yupiit have achieved *partial* recognition of their ability to manage Yup'ik child welfare. Representatives from the Yup'ik nonprofit are invited to attend and comment on child custody court cases involving Yup'ik children and are included in the discussions with lawyers and Office of Children's Services representatives in which expectations for caregivers' treatment are established.

Despite these inclusions, Linda lamented the degree to which her organization's input was frequently disregarded. She described one particularly troubling case involving a twelve-year-old boy who was in the process of being adopted by nonnative parents living outside the region. As the adoption became imminent, the boy began asking questions: Why hadn't his grandmother adopted him? Would his mother approve of the adoption if she knew that his adoptive parents were nonnative?

Linda's nonprofit talked to the boy's soon-to-be-adoptive parents and invited them to attend Healing Our Families, which covers issues of native identity and Yup'ik heritage. Although the adoptive parents were interested in attending, the Office of Children's Services refused to allow the boy to participate. The Office's representatives claimed that the workshop would cause emotional harm to the boy and questioned whether Linda's nonprofit was, as Linda put it, "equipped to handle his reactions." They expressed their doubts about whether Linda and her colleagues had a plan for addressing the boy's response to the workshop, suggesting that they had not fully thought through the ramifications of their invitation. In this and other cases the state of Alaska's representatives denied the competence of Yup'ik leadership, refusing to recognize the legitimacy of the methods that Yupiit have developed for addressing complex emotional issues.

The form of recognition that was denied to Yupiit leadership in this instance shades into a related form of recognition: the way states' claims to sovereignty are substantiated through formal or informal *recognition* of their legitimacy from other states. In the United States recognition of this form usually refers to the federal government's explicit acknowledgment of the sovereign status of a particular Native American tribe, as established by the Bureau of Indian Affairs through the Federal Acknowledgment Process (Miller 2004). This declaration of recognition is founded on a judgment of the tribe's *legitimacy*, based on criteria established by the federal government.[19] Yet recognition of native sovereignty is not necessarily an all-or-nothing phenomenon, and it may involve other players (Cattelino 2008; Howland and White 2009; Miller 2004). As Cattelino illustrates for the Florida Seminole, sovereignty is built up through relationships of interdependency between native and nonnative governments, in which acknowledgments of legitimacy are both reciprocal and implied. Howland and White (2009: 12) further note that the legitimacy of *any* polity is conferred not by a single state but by an international community. This may be doubly true for indigenous polities. With the passing of the United Nations Declarations of the Rights of Indigenous Peoples in 2007, native groups may increasingly be looking toward a global sovereign to instantiate their claims to legitimacy (Millon 2013).

What I mean to suggest is that everyday recognitions of the legitimacy of Yup'ik leadership together instantiate Yup'ik claims to sovereignty. This brings us back to the issue of metrics. The state of Alaska joins multiple national and transnational institutions in adopting quantitative evidence of efficacy as a precondition for the recognition of the legitimacy of health programs. Without health metrics to back it up, Healing Our Families may be unable to achieve legitimacy from either the Office of Children's Services or the multiplicity of national and transnational entities that together constitute the world of global health. And without such legitimacy, recognition — in its multiple registers — becomes a distant dream.

Evidence at Any Cost

We might nonetheless ask: Are the forms of recognition afforded by participation in the production of health metrics worth their cost? The creation of programs such as Principles of Health and Healing Our Families suggests that Yupiit are prioritizing the revitalization of local knowledge. Many believe that this knowledge holds the key to overcoming the behavioral health issues that the region now faces. The use of health metrics may undermine these recent efforts to affirm the legitimacy of local knowledge.

Health metrics are purported to be objective measures that are universally applicable, and they are fast becoming a precondition for state and private funding. Yet health metrics are the products of a particular kind of technical, rational, secular scientific knowledge that contrasts with Yup'ik formulations of knowledge involving the inseparability of the spiritual from the natural, the legitimacy of intuitive understandings, and the im-

portance of elders' unique expertise. The Yup'ik anthropologist Oscar Kawagley (2006) makes note of this when he critiques the purported universality of Western science. Kawagley points out that the Yup'ik worldview
does not maintain a distinction between belief and knowledge. Both empirical observations and intuitive experiences are valid foundations for
understanding. While statistical measures of efficacy are purported to be
universally applicable, they are premised on a rational scientific worldview
that contrasts with Yup'ik wisdom. Health metrics may thus end up under-
cutting the very sovereignty they are meant to protect, potentially altering
the "self" over which "self-governance" is sought.

Furthermore, when the provision of health services is made conditional
on the production of new kinds of quantitative evaluation criteria, the
kinds of programs that can be offered may be limited. As Linda and Sally
suggested, not all modes of healing can be isolated and quantified. The
introduction of health metrics today seems to be about how to count outcomes, but the very language of statistical evaluation tends to restrict what
kinds of evidence come to *count* as outcomes at all.

This challenge was brought to my attention during an interview with my
friend Ellen, a middle-aged Yup'ik woman who works in another branch of
the native nonprofit. Ellen discussed the healing dimensions of subsistence
practices, such as subsistence salmon fishing, that Yup'ik people rely on:

It's not just "gathering." The process of subsistence fishing means we
have to get together and get along. It's just something we do. This
time of year is the only time I'll see my sister Elena and my mom and
be together. It forces us to work together, and so we open up and we
start talking. A lot of times it's like filling an emotional void. It's that
one time when we have to face up to each other. We're working right
next to each other, and there's no secrets.

You know, when I sobered up, I had gone to this treatment center
in Washington. And part of the treatment is [that] my husband and
my mom had to go in and have treatment with me, because they're
major players in my life. And my husband stopped drinking when
he went. My mom, she never drank in her life, never smoked, she
doesn't swear. She's a preacher's kid, and in a good way. She said,
"You've drifted far from me." And she said, "You drank, and you're
not the same person." She said, "The way to get healthy is [for] you
[to] come back and do your thing. Let's start going back to fishcamp

together. Let's start working together." And she said, "You need that! That's your therapy." . . .

So it's spiritual. You know, you get your fish, but it's way more than that. It's a lifestyle, it's reaffirming what we do and what we like, what we are.

Ellen considered subsistence practices to be a form of "treatment" that helped her recover from addiction. Yet the healing power of subsistence fishing cannot be isolated from its many other functions. As Ellen pointed out, subsistence fishing is simultaneously a form of manual labor, a mode of sociality, an instantiation of kinship ties, a spiritual practice, and an emotional affirmation. As Kawagley (2006) predicts, multiple dimensions of human experience are interwoven in the practice of subsistence fishing, and a single thread cannot be pulled out. This understanding of interconnectedness is built into the model of healthy living articulated in Yup'ik behavioral health rubrics. But they are not easily captured in the kind of metrics that funders want. Isolating practices in ways that can be held constant from client to client, clinic to clinic, health indicator to health indicator was antithetical to the approach of Yup'ik behavioral health programs. Yet there is evidence to suggest that these programs are already being pushed in this direction.

Fidelity to the Model

I returned to Tundra Flats shortly after the three-year grant period for Healing Our Families had drawn to a close. Linda's nonprofit had succeeded in securing another four years of funding for the program from the same granting agency. But the agency had dramatically restructured the grant to follow a data-driven framework, and Linda was unsure how her nonprofit would meet the new expectations outlined in the grant. She and her colleagues were now required to follow a five-step procedure that would guide them through the creation and implementation of an evidence-based behavioral health intervention. Grantees were required to purchase a computer software system that would allow them to develop logic models to evaluate the potential effectiveness of their proposed program. After completing each step, grantees would be evaluated according to a "fidelity checklist" that would assess the degree to which they had adhered to the outlined procedure. The granting agency representative leading the orientation for new grantees suggested that renewal of funding might be influenced by the grantees' fidelity to the model. She also stressed that grantees would not be permitted to proceed to the next step in the process until they had satisfied the essential checklist items.

The purportedly apolitical language of quantitative evidence masks the post/colonial power dynamics at play here. The legitimacy of Yup'ik behavioral health programs has been denied, and Linda and her colleagues' expert knowledge of Yup'ik principles of wellness has been discounted. As a grant recipient, Linda's nonprofit must choose *one* behavioral health issue to be working under, such as suicide prevention, substance abuse, or mental health. This fragmentation of health services is a far cry from Ellen's description of the therapeutic value of subsistence fishing as an integrative process. Furthermore, the conditions of the grant dictate that Linda's nonprofit must build the behavioral health intervention from scratch based on evidence of efficacy that they are being compelled to collect and report. Linda told me with a sigh that they would have to spend their whole first year on data collection and planning, despite the fact that the curriculum for Healing Our Families had been developed and refined over the course of almost six years.

Linda did not appear to be the only one frustrated by these new stipulations. During an informational webinar provided by the granting agency, another grantee raised the following question: "Obviously, we've very committed to going through the [data-driven] process, and looking forward to it. If, however, there is an implementation opportunity that arises early in the process that might be time sensitive, and if the coalition believes that that implementation opportunity is one that we should [pursue], is there any opportunity to use the implementation funds before our plan is done, or is that a bright line?" Although this grantee affirmed the value of the data-driven process, she questioned the necessity of strictly adhering to the outlined procedure. Surely there was some room to adapt to changing circumstances, particularly if there was consensus among the local leadership on the value of an intervention. But the granting agency representative's response suggests a different set of priorities: "That's a pretty bright line. And the reason is that, if we do that, then we start not having *fidelity to the process*. Because basically what that's saying is, you haven't finished the process, but you've already selected a strategy. So, with these funds, it's going to be very important that strategies are not started until after you've completed the process."

Underlying this dispute over the importance of "fidelity to the model" is a deeper debate about what must be done differently to finally alleviate the persistent emotional suffering of Yup'ik people. For Yup'ik leaders such as Linda, the ongoing conditions of post/colonial occupation are responsible for the behavioral health struggles that Yupiit face today. The decades of "treatment" that have been provided to Yupiit have failed to improve behavioral health outcomes because they have failed to address the root causes of emotional distress. If anything, such "treatments" have contributed to the post/colonial conditions that perpetuate distress (Stevenson 2014). The solution therefore involves reclaiming responsibility for the provision of vital services from state and federal governments, asserting the validity of local knowledge and expertise in the process. In other words, it both requires and instantiates Yup'ik sovereignty.

For the federal, state, and private granting agencies that fund Yup'ik behavioral health programs, the answers lie elsewhere. Decades of failed behavioral health interventions have been ineffective because they didn't have the right tools. Previous programs didn't collect baseline health information or measure effectiveness. They didn't quantify the impact of their interventions to determine which should be continued and which should be abandoned. As Adams (chapter 1, this volume) points out, everything that came before the introduction of quantitative evidence criteria is rendered suspect.

Today, Yup'ik leaders and behavioral health workers are finding innovative ways around the limitations placed on them by federal, state, and private granting agencies. They are engaging creatively with health metrics and making metrics work for them, both in their immediate efforts to promote Yup'ik wellness and in their broader struggles for Yup'ik sovereignty. I have no doubt that they are up to the challenge. Yet we must ask ourselves about the value of statistical measures of efficacy in post/colonial contexts in which indigenous groups are fighting for the right to have their own understandings of wellness count in global health.

Notes

1. All names have been changed, including the name of the town and its institutions of health care and governance.

2. In 2013 I spent eleven weeks doing participant-observation in Tundra Flats's public health nursing center, accompanying the nurses as they went about their daily tasks.

I attended multiple public and semiprivate meetings with nursing staff and attended three trainings offered by local social service agencies. I also spent time in five nearby villages, including a three-day business trip with one of the itinerant public health nurses and a week-long visit with a friend's extended family in a different village. I returned to Tundra Flats in 2014 for an additional six weeks of participant-observation and follow-up with several indigenous social service organizations and health programs.

3. My use of the term *behavioral health* throughout this essay reflects the common health parlance of the region, where it is used by native and nonnative residents alike to refer to mental and emotional health as well as behaviors such as substance use, interpersonal and interpartner violence, child abuse and neglect, self-harm, and suicide.

4. I use the term *indigenous* here in order to draw a connection between the contested status of native peoples in the United States and the contested status of native peoples elsewhere. Otherwise I use *native* and *indigenous* interchangeably.

5. There is a rich literature in Native American Studies that interrogates the meaning and value of self-governance. Deloria and Lytle (1984) point out that self-government is a foreign concept that was pushed onto Native American tribes in order to facilitate management by the federal government. Simpson (2014) questions what it means for the U.S. settler-state to confer sovereignty when it was responsible for robbing Native American tribes of inherent sovereign rights. Without diminishing the significance of these critiques, for the purposes of this essay I presume the value of self-governance in order to put Yup'ik struggles for sovereignty in conversation with transnational global health trends.

6. Quote from Adams, ch. 1, this volume. My use of punctuation in the term *post/colonial* is influenced by Loomba 2005.

7. I have largely avoided using the term *tribe* to describe Alaska Native groups, as this is a particularly slippery term in the Alaskan context. As Huhndorf and Huhndorf (2011: 398) explain, "In the Alaskan context, *tribes* is usually synonymous with *villages*, which have traditionally been self-governing, autonomous units, and the list of federally recognized tribes in Alaska is villages. Villages have social, cultural, and linguistic affiliations with broader entities (Tlingit, Athabaskan, Yup'ik, and so on) that are sometimes also called tribes, especially for purposes of self-identification."

8. Twelve of the for-profit regional native corporations own property within a geographic region whose residents roughly correspond to a shared linguistic group. The thirteenth corporation includes Alaska Natives who did not live in the state of Alaska at the time ANCSA was signed into law. Village corporations can adopt for-profit or nonprofit status. Nonprofit village corporations provide community services rather than distribute dividends.

9. Subsequent amendments have allowed corporations to extend enrollment to natives born after 1971 if they so choose (Linxwiler 2007).

10. Since the passing of ANCSA, Alaska Natives have sought to shore up legislation to ensure that native corporations continue to operate as tribal entities. A 1988 amendment restricts the selling of stock indefinitely, and thus far no ANCSA corporation has made stock available for outside purchase.

11. *Tribe* is a problematic term for Native American groups as well as for Alaska Native peoples. Miller (2004: 8) points out, "Much of the controversy surrounding the acknowledgement process centers upon the fact that there is simply no agreement on what a 'tribe' is, and therefore there is little consensus on how to recognize one."

12. The status of American Indian tribes is diverse. Many tribes did not sign treaties with the federal government or have not had their treaties legally affirmed and therefore remain "unrecognized." For more on Native American sovereignty, see, for example, Deloria and Lytle 1984.

13. Governmentality is a concept drawn from the work of Foucault (see especially 2003, 2007, 2008).

14. In official publications and everyday conversations behavioral health program directors most often use the terms *traditional knowledge, cultural knowledge,* or *Yup'ik knowledge.* I instead use the term *local knowledge* (Foucault 2003) to preserve the contrast between these forms of knowledge and hegemonic notions of expertise, while at the same time avoiding the suggestion that "tradition," "culture," or "tribal" affiliation is a unique, necessary, and enduring feature of *native* groups specifically (Povinelli 2006).

15. To preserve the anonymity of the organization and its directors, I have not included citations to the organization's website, where many of these primary source documents can be found. References can be provided on a per-request basis.

16. For more on historical trauma, see the work of Brave Heart (especially 2004). For an incisive critique of the therapeutic theory of trauma in indigenous communities, see Millon (2013).

17. The health corporation is a cosigner to the Alaska Tribal Health Compact, a consortium that negotiates annual funding agreements with the Indian Health Service for federal funds designated for health care services to Alaska Natives.

18. The policy of self-determination adopted by the federal government in the 1970s is arguably also an assimilationist policy (see Deloria and Lytle 1984). I do not mean to throw my own support behind self-determination as a rubric for relations with native groups, but only to point out the hypocrisy of these structures of financial dependency and to hold the federal government accountable to its own stated policies.

19. It is disturbing that a branch of the federal government is considered the final arbiter in judging the legitimacy of Native American tribes.

PART III. METRICS ECONOMICS

6 · METRICS AND MARKET LOGICS OF GLOBAL HEALTH

SUSAN L. ERIKSON

We are moving out of an era when governments alone are expected to fix local health problems, and we are at an unruly historical moment in health care provision worldwide. Can the market take care of everything? Mid-nineteenth-century governance reforms in Bismarck's Germany and Chadwick's England catalyzed global expectations that nation-states should pay for, organize, and provide health services. These sensibilities informed both colonizing and colonized states in a variety of ways, but the expectation itself began to wane with the mid-twentieth-century rise of neoliberal economic policies requiring nation-state pullback and business promotion in newly independent states. Into this void international bankers, business executives, and some heads of state marched market logics. Even as some people still hold to the idea of state-centric delivery of primary health services, anthropologists attest to the multitudes and variabilities of health services lash-ups—public, private, and in combination—in the twenty-first century (e.g., Adams 2013b; Livingston 2012; Van Hollen 2013). Throughout the world organizing principles of pastoral health care are giving way to speculative, market-driven ideas of health (Dumit 2012; Rajan 2012), prompting and being prompted by new global health investment instruments desperately in need of metrics. Beyond old-style accountability, metrics create *value* in these new global health investment schematics.

Accountability metrics still feature significantly in global health programming, as is well documented in this volume. But there is a new shadow life to numbers in global health as well: numbers are needed not just to account for money spent, to gauge program impact, or to evaluate health outcomes — those are retrospective metrics — but also to make future *actuarial* worth. The shift from accountability metrics to "value" metrics is a shift to prospective future-centric value. This shift to value arises at a time when "a defining quality of our current moment is its characteristic state of anticipation" (Adams et al. 2009: 246). Multiple global health actors are taking up market logics with an "excited forward looking" (247) in which "the future is what matters most" (248). Using metrics as anticipatory praxis means that global health commodities like drugs, medical devices, water engineering, and care itself are assessed in terms of not only people's health outcomes but also how much money they are likely to make for investors in the future.

Numerical health indicators are inextricable metrics of our times (Erikson 2015a; Wendland, this volume). Such accountability metrics have been with us for several decades, as Adams (chapter 1, this volume) notes and Smith-Morris (this volume) fleshes out. Increasingly, though, accountability metrics are becoming tethered to market metrics and logics, which is the focus of my chapter. I primarily draw from two geographical sites: Sierra Leone, where I worked for two years as an international development worker before its war (1991–2002) and where I now conduct research as an anthropologist, and Washington, DC, where I worked for U.S. government international development agencies. Further I draw from recent interviews and conversations with people living and working in global finance in Vancouver, British Columbia; Seattle, Washington; and New York City, as well as from research from cyber and digital sites where the machinations of global health finance are in evidence. These differently constituted sites, incommensurable in many ways, nonetheless enable analyses of global health as a worldwide social field within which health likelihoods are mutually constituted through relations of power (Erikson 2008).

Central to understanding the underlying principles of new forms of global health financing are two basic premises: global health commodities like drugs, medical devices, and water technologies are both (1) goods in which to invest with the expectation of making more money and (2) objects "lashed up" (Murray Li 2005) with financial instruments, corporate moneymaking, and government policy incentives. I've become increasingly interested in the demonstrably variable notions of investment and return on investment, especially the different kinds of profits and yields claimed by differently positioned people working in the ever emergent social field of global health. Describing the need to appeal to greed when he sold investors on social impact investing, a term used to signal concurrence of beneficial social change with financial return to investors, one financial advisor said, "They don't have to have good motives to do good things.... Our whole mission is to get global health investors to stay in it because they are going to make money. I don't trust anybody's motives simply on the basis of being good!" In health, a field where altruistic claims and high notions of common good are commonplace, the cohabitation of ideas about good and innocence, avarice and esurience are analytically compelling.

Shift from Accountability Metrics

Statistics—their production, circulation, application, and control—have long played important roles in exercises of power within nation-states. My anthropological interest in banal hegemonic power structures prompted questions about how statistics work *between* nation-states. I started thinking about the new powers people afforded statistics during a 2008 trip to Sierra Leone. In 2005 the Gates Foundation had invested $US50 million in seed money for a health information system in five pilot countries, one of which was Sierra Leone. As a result statistical collection, aggregation, and application in postconflict Sierra Leone (the war officially ended in 2002) was led for some time by health and humanitarian sectors. In 2012, with funding from the Social Science and Humanities Research Council of Canada, I began a research project in Sierra Leone to study how health statistics moved between the health, humanitarian, and commercial sectors, tracing exchanges and outcomes as prewar 1960 models of government-to-government overseas development aid were replaced by an "unruly mélange" (Buse and Walt 1997) of largely private donor money, competing provisioners, philanthropic ambitions, and venture capitalism. Half of Sierra Leone's national operating budget today comes from outside sources, and the use of statistics, often to make decisions "at a distance" (Latour 1987), play an important role in this budget.

Statistical information and sector-specific indicators are the shorthand references that business investors and public sector policymakers believe are critical to decision making. Since the early 2000s one of the key players in global health, the Bill and Melinda Gates Foundation, has developed significant, far-reaching statistical systems to better audit global health. The Institute for Health Metrics and Evaluation (IHME) in Seattle and the Health Metrics Network in Geneva are two of the Gates Foundation's early protégés funded to achieve that goal. About five years ago, however, the singular focus on numbers-for-audit, deployed for the accountability of global health outcomes, expanded to include a focus on numbers-for-investment. Financial institutions and investment banks took due notice. Jamie Dimon, chairman of the board of directors and chief executive officer of JPMorgan Chase and Co., said, "The Gates Foundation, one of the things it's done, probably *the* most impactful thing is, they are bringing discipline, math, analytics and science to philanthropy in a way that's never been done before" (Global Health Investment Fund [GHIF] 2013).

The money the Gates Foundation has given to create statistical systems the world over has produced multiple dividends, not least of which now includes those for the financial sector. Statistical health metrics inform humanitarian networks and restructure how public goods like health are governed. Increasingly they also inform capital markets. Statistics, as a knowledge technology, travels globally, from resource-rich countries to resource-poor countries and back, and back, and back, in keeping with Latour's (1987) "centers of calculation," all the while being put to multiple ends. Financial advisors hired by the Gates Foundation, work hard to sell the simple idea that "you can make money doing good things." One told me, "Investors will want to accomplish good things once they see they can make money." Another told me, "We are harnessing a value-creation machine . . . [in a] sort of twilight zone where the land of darkness and the land of light overlaps."

Humanitarian and commercial endeavors had been more separate in decades past, but statistics now enable these domains to operate in mutually constitutive ways. In Sierra Leone, although data production and statistical analysis are policy imperatives of the government, the maturity of data sets is uneven between social sectors. The health sector has one of the most established data sets. Investment portfolios for mining and other private-sector ventures often include health statistics as one of the few hard data sources appearing regularly.

By the Numbers: Incentivizing Global Health

A primary argument driving new financial arrangements in global health is that moneymaking—and *only* moneymaking—will motivate people to fix global health problems. Bill Gates spoke for an entire group of people when he noted in his 2013 Annual Letter, "Tool[s] of business [will] improve the health and welfare of more of the world's people." Anthropologists have long been interested in tools and technologies used to get a job done; in global health, health metrics are among the tools this new generation of global health investors are talking about. Incentivizing financial technologies are vast, running the gamut from simple spreadsheets to complex derivatives. The development of increasingly complex financial incentives for investing in global health—as a "thing," asset, commodity—has been fomenting in earnest for almost a decade.

Among those early innovators were Aidan Hollis and Thomas Pogge (2008), who, beginning in the early 2000s, gained some attention and initially some traction when they proposed a "market-based solution" to develop medicines for neglected diseases experienced primarily by poor people. Their Health Impact Fund (HIF) schema promised to "revolutionize health outcomes" by rewarding pharmaceutical companies for distributing medicines at cost. Governments would provide the initial investments, many millions to start. The reward system Hollis and Pogge envisioned was problematic from the start, however. Pogge, who continues to be HIF's most ardent public champion, believed rather simplistically that better drugs would get better outcomes in all scenarios, that pharmaceutical companies would compete for the best outcomes, that competition would produce better results, and that on-the-ground context did not matter much. His plan was that the HIF would reward companies investing in neglected disease treatments with a simple comparison between test subjects who had taken the new drug and subjects who had not taken the drug. Quality-adjusted life years (QALY)—a number quantifying improved wellness resulting from a health treatment or intervention—was a primary measure of a treatment's success for these two test groups. Interest started strong, but it dissipated.

Pogge's model offers an interesting moment of transition between nonprofit public- and for-profit private-sector funding for health. Initially he called for investments from governments, but only insofar as these would spawn the private sector's commitment to health programs that might generate profits. He recommended that governments contribute .03 percent of their gross national income to start this fund. This amounted to a standing fund of about $US6 billion, which introduced a number of problems for the fund right from the start. As is the case with the World Bank and the International Monetary Fund, the United States by virtue of the size of its gross national income would be putting more money in than all other countries. Proportionate U.S. control over assessments could have been anticipated since the promise of fiscal rewards is tied to them. One of the weakest parts of the HIF plan, in fact, was its failure to think critically about the measurement systems that would adjudicate the annual financial returns. Pogge (2010, personal communication) placed blind acceptance in measurement systems known to be fraught with controversy (e.g., Mortimer and Segal 2008; Schlander 2010).

Pogge's entreaties were concurrent with the global recession in 2008 and after. During that time wealthy people the world over were continuing to make money on investments despite the economic downturn, which was (and continues to be) experienced primarily by the middle and working classes.[1] Income increases for the rich came predominantly not from wage labor but from investment capital returns. "High-wealth individuals," as investors are known, bankrolled new technologies, commodities, and companies in a multitude of new sectors, including the global health sector. Social impact investing is increasingly popular (Sullivan 2014) and picks up where Hollis and Pogge left off. The HIF design begged money from governments, but the latest round of global health investment incentives are being promoted by global health foundations, individual investors, and private corporations.

One area of investor interest has been global health research and development, which during the past several years been touted as a moneymaker by global investment forecasters. Research and development is an investment category savvy investors understand; put your money in now, while a health treatment, medical device, or drug is developed, and cash in your return after it hits the market. This meshing of global health "good" with moneymaking is not new; it is especially well-established in the pharmaceutical industry (Dumit 2012; Peterson 2014; Petryna 2009). But the number of investments is both increasing and diversifying as devices and technologies come together in new ways (e.g., ultrasound and cell phones). More frequently now nonprofits like public health–oriented Population Services International (PSI) and trade association–derived BIO Ventures for Global Health (BVGH) actively promote private-sector investments in global health research. Publications, such as PSI's *Impact* "Best Buys Issue: Where to Invest in Global Health 2014" (2014), and annual conventions, such as the Global Event for Biotechnology, sponsored by the Biotechnology Industry Organization (BIO) tout new devices and technologies in which to invest. Similarly, Adams (chapter 1, this volume) notes the growth of moneymaking on instruments for doing global health research as "toolkits" become necessary for both doing evidence-based interventions and managing the research data they generate.

BIO is a particularly interesting example of how the nonprofit arms of corporations provide some cover for profit-making strategies. Organizations like BIO sponsor big conventions designed to bring new product inventors in contact with investors with deep pockets. The BIO-sponsored panel session for the 2011 Partnering for Global Health Forum featured four panelists from JPMorgan, the financial services firm; a drug-discovery company; a drug and diagnostics development company; and BVGH.[2] The former three panelists are all for-profit entities; the BVGH officer was the lone official nonprofit representative, with the industry connections described earlier. In the panel discussion global health was touted as one of the few arenas in 2011 where investors could expect annual returns of 10 percent or better—a stunning claim considering that such profits were rare since the 2008 global financial downturn. A significant portion of the panel discussion was devoted to global health as an investment, complete with recommendations of developing country-specific investments and predictions of expected growth, that is, how much money could be made per place and commodity. The discussion exemplifies a new kind of global health, in which investment by the very rich with an expectation and anticipation of return on investments is considered optimal for achieving health.

It is not hard to uncover that the nonprofit BVGH — "whose mission is to save lives" (according to their website) — is tightly linked to a parent company, Biotechnology Industry Organization. The board of directors for BVGH is populated by present and former BIO executives. Observers might call BVGH the "friendly" arm of the BIO, which is a biotech trade organization based in Washington, DC. BIO's lobbying efforts are pro-corporation, promoting the biotech commodities of their members. In November 2013, for example, their efforts included lobbying in the United States against government-organized health care and against a Washington state law requiring the labeling of genetically engineered foods, the logic being that government-organized health care and labeling amounted to market interference.

Lobbying associations like BIO represent the interests of biotechnology corporations by lobbying for public policies and subsidies that support the use and consumption of the products that are produced by the corporations who support them. Such organizations are nothing new; neither is government support for these organizations. (I worked with U.S. government programs designed to support just such trade organizations in the 1980s.) Trade associations have long set up offices in capital cities to influence public policies in ways that are favorable to corporate sales. What has changed over the past several decades is the degree to which global health and other human welfare endeavors have become user-friendly *investment* vehicles. Less than a generation ago, health, education, and other social welfare sectors were considered zero-profit sectors, often operating at a deficit (there were some exceptions, like pharmaceutical companies). Arguably there was an implicit social consensus that it was necessary for every federal government to subsidize health, education, and welfare sectors (the so-called safety net). Today the shift to anticipatory market logics and for-profit opportunism is pervasive in all three sectors. At a 2014 social impact forum, Jason Saul (2014), CEO of Mission Measurement, a business management consultant group, put it this way: "[Before], accountability demanded different measurement. Accountability basically said, 'How do you prove that you're not wasting my money? I need to see about your metrics. I need an audit.' Today, the questions are different. . . . Which outcomes can you produce for me? . . . What is your relative cost per outcome compared to everybody else? What is my expected yield from my investment in your charity?" Anticipating outcomes requires different metrics than accountability reporting, which brings us, again, to the ways metrics are essential to enumerating value.

Making Future Value, Literally

A prospective emphasis on outcomes requires a fundamental change in health metrics, which have been proposed retrospectively for a very long time. To get investors to invest, value must be convertible to cash. In global health this has meant that the primary question of how to calculate value had to change from "Did the person get better after such and such treatment?" to "What is the probability that such and such a treatment can be sold in the future?" With this calculative shift, financial advisors began coaching global health foundations and directing them toward new investment domains. A financial advisor to global health foundations told me, "About five years ago, [philanthropic global health foundations] wanted to see what they could do in international development spaces as targets of investment, and I went to work for them because this space has the potential to be cash flow–positive, it's investable! There was no one helping them to see the investment opportunity there!"

Convincing investors to invest in global health commodities means elaborating value. A Vancouver financial analyst told me jovially, "Value? How do we get it? Well, we make it!" I was conducting an interview in his enormous, well-appointed modern kitchen, when I asked him to explain what he meant when he said, "That company had no value." "What was value?" I asked, and he answered, "Value is an estimate of how much money the company can generate *in the future* [my emphasis]. It is a well-informed estimate, I have to say. But it gets used in all kinds of ways, even in divorce settlements, the wife wants to know how much the company is worth so she can get alimony!"

When I asked him to describe what he *does* to get value, he answered in an avuncular way. "I sit myself down in that chair in my office, get all my monitors going with news, and reports, and stock numbers, I read through it all and write a recommendation. It can take a while."

Different analysts make value with different ingredients. Social and political events can affect value, as Stefan Leins (2011) describes in "Pricing the Revolution," about Egypt's January 2011 revolution impact on valuations. A Seattle mining analyst I interviewed factors in the quality of ore based on geological drill samples he himself collects on visits to extraction sites around the world. (Earlier in his career he had overvalued a gold mining company that had no gold.) Site visits like his, as it turns out, are uncommon—most valuations are done in front of a computer—but this Seattle analyst's reputation for traveling to "the ends of the earth" (which included Sierra Leone) garnered him a die-another-day bravado and kudos from his fellow analysts.

Making value depends on multiple variables, moving across time and space. "Doing the math" simplifies. "Complexity made it difficult to decide where value lay, and thus opened the door to mathematically adept modellers on [Wall] Street" (Derman 2004: 120). Most of the analysts I interviewed made a point of saying that they did not always use numeric formulas in lockstep, but the vast majority described familiarity with using the formulas to calculate relationships between standard Wall Street variables. Since the 1980s, in fact, computer software has been available to do the math—to code equations and process numerical data. One classic valuation model is the Gordon Growth Model (Gordon and Shapiro 1956), which is still used in its original and iterative forms:

$$Value\ (P) = Dividend\ (D)\ /\ Return\ (k) - Growth\ (G)$$

Beyond valuation, another formula, the Weighted Average Cost of Capital WACC (Miles and Ezzell 1980), helps investors decide what the minimum returns need to be to make their investment worthwhile:

$$WACC = kE + (1{-}t)\ rD\ /\ D + E$$

"where E, D, k, and r denote equity, debt, the cost of equity, and the interest rate on debt" (Arzac 1986:123). The point here is not to debate or even explain any of these equations (there are hundreds more), as business school professors might, but rather to show that financiers use quantitative formulas to determine value. Numbers—indicators, accountability, and actuarial numbers—are used in conjunction with these equations to make value.

What has intensified in the past decade is the demand for quantifying social domains previously believed incommensurable with market opportunities. But, as Rajan (2012) and Dumit (2012) note, quantifying value through equations like this can be far removed from calculating whether or not goods actually make people healthier. How one calibrates health outcomes in relation to fiscal returns is nowhere more complicated than in the work of the Gates Foundation.

In 2014, five years after financial advisors began prompting foundations to use investment instruments in global health, Bill Gates again became a flag bearer for promoting financial investment logics through philanthrocapitalism in global health. In a promotional video for a new fund, the Global Health Investment Fund, which partnered the Gates Foundation with the investment bank JPMorgan Chase and others, Gates said, "Global health, although it seems like the hardest kind of philanthropy [relative to return on investment], really . . . it's actually in my view one of the low risk forms of philanthropy" (GHIF 2014). By "low risk," he explains, the money given by investors has a high chance of producing a return on investment. He means "return" in two ways: one is in the form of documentable "good"; the other means—and he is speaking to wealthy potential investors here—you have a low risk of losing money if you invest with this fund. He goes on to use the words *investment* and *philanthropy* interchangeably and makes clear that this form of philanthropy includes not just giving money away but also getting money back. In fact its architects suggest that it will provide a 5 to 7 percent return on investment.[3]

There is a discursive slippage in this language. Investments *for* making money and investments *of* time and effort to improve health have not always been synonymous. In these new investment schematics, however, epidemiological health risks are flattened so that they can be used in the service of determining investment risk. A new goal for foundations is to work with investment banks to get investors (large net-worth individuals) on board with making money on early ("upstream") product development (e.g., vaccine development and other commodities that require a long-term investment). In time, the logic goes, large distributions of vaccines will result in financial profit. The departure from traditional philanthropy outcomes is that now foundations will be tracking two outcomes, financial and health, which can be mutually exclusive, as Rajan (2012) and Dumit (2012) document so well. One outcome does not guarantee the other. It is entirely possible that money can be made on vaccine development even if its disease is not prevented or reduced, as many investors already know.

Corporate social responsibility, a term used since the 1960s to signal socially beneficial contributions made by corporations, is newly defined in partnerships like the GHIF. Corporate philanthropy is no longer simply about giving money away; it is about making money in the same way these companies and their executives always have, for themselves, their causes, and their shareholders (Erikson 2015b). Susanne Craig posits an additional return benefit in her *New York Times* essay, "Goldman Sachs, Buying Redemption," noting that philanthropic motivations also include a "reputational return,"[4] one accomplished through metrics.

Following the Money

Metrics are needed to *make* actuarial worth in the investment worlds of global health. In the process value gets enumerated and assigned a monetary equivalence. Health is also assigned value in these equations, and metrics make health values correspond to financial values. When social scientists follow the money in the worlds of global health finance we increasingly find that health has become a thing en route to, amid, and alongside making money. Health must become, in other words, a fungible "thing," a movable part. Health signs and symbols — indicators, for example — enumerate and as a result are available as investment factors capable of being plugged into investment equations. In fact fungibility is required of global health and global health "products" in order for them to become investment worthy; profitable health commodities can ideally be cashed out at any time. Investors need to be able to anticipate this outcome — the point at which their investment can be cashed in as money in their accounts. These new conduits for financial investment are believed by some to be absolutely essential for improving health and reducing human suffering.

Consider what many transnational businesses are comfortable calling "reverse innovation" (Govindarajan and Trimble 2012; Immelt et al. 2009). The "trickle-up" effect discussed by Gates in describing the GHIF requires transnational companies to coax good ideas to "flow uphill" (Govindarajan 2012), often by throwing money at the innovators in impoverished geographies. Reverse innovation — the begging, borrowing, buying, and sometimes stealing of ideas and technology from the so-called Global South for use in the so-called Global North — is grounded in global corporations' newly found recognition that the Global South is home to great, and lucrative, ideas and applications, some of which are in the health sector.

When we move into contemporary and emerging domains of global health finance and investment, we find that the conventional nation-state geographies of global public health do not work well enough to fully explain how money moves or how it is made. Money does not stay within the bounded political territories of nation-states used by, among others, the World Health Organization and international diplomatic corps. While the world is not as flat as Thomas Friedman would have us believe, moving money transnationally has gotten significantly easier since 1989, and this has made fundamental differences to how health funding is governed. Moving and making money were both made easier with the 1995 passage of the World Trade Organization's General Agreement on Trade and Services (GATS) (Sexton 2003) that, in effect, made health a fungible commodity. Prior to GATS most services (health, education, welfare) had been widely deemed public services for the public good, often provisioned by governments, and discernibly not for profit. After GATS, health, education, and welfare services became legally categorized as global commercial enterprises. Such a reconceptualization of basic safety-net services has been taken up in various ways by various nation-states, but the overall trend for business has meant an increase in global investment "instruments," "arrangements," and capital market "solutions" using health goods and services as things that can be traded across national boundaries with ease.

This is not to say that global health finance is the same everywhere. Jane Guyer (2004) and Bill Maurer (2013) are right about the variabilities of economic valuation, acquisition, and accumulation throughout the world; there are many ways to create economic value, meaning, and exchange. Still, opening up global markets to invest in safety-net activities, like health and health care in poor countries, has led to some strange bedfellow investments. Some foundations have been taken to task for "growing" money by investing in businesses that seem at cross purposes with expressed charitable missions. For example, in 2000 the *New York Times* reported that the Gates Foundation was giving money away to the American Cancer Society at the same time it held bonds in the tobacco giant Philip Morris.[5] In 2007 the *Los Angeles Times* published a series of articles based on ninety interviews and hundreds of documents, including many from the Gates Foundation itself as well as the U.S. Securities and Exchange Commission. Among the most damning articles in the series—and the one that provoked the strongest response from the Gates Foundation and supporters— was one entitled "Dark Cloud over Good Works of Gates Foundation."[6] This article prompted Amy Goodman and *DemocracyNow!* to write "Gates Foundation Causing Harm with the Same Money It Uses to Do Good."[7] In 2011 Stuckler et al. (2011) reported on Gates board members owning shares in and profiting from gains by some of the same companies that public health professionals fight with about aggressive corporate marketing campaigns and links to downturns in public health. Others have taken the Gates Foundation to task for profiting from their shares in Coca-Cola, McDonald's, and Monsanto (Global Health Watch 2011).

What is the problem here? Are there downsides to financing global health using the same mechanisms one would use to run an investment portfolio? In many ways it is too early to know, and we can expect huge variability in the effect and outcomes of these tactics around the world. I need to regularly remind myself that not every country has the same configuration of challenges seen in Sierra Leone. But it is important at this point to take note of these new trends in global health finance and to try to trace their effects in all senses of the term. Adams (2013b) charted how market logics superseded vital social services provision after a natural disaster, concluding as well that the charity and philanthrocapitalism that are now used "for taking care of those in need" get caught up in the same eddies of profit making (at the expense of service provision) that for-profit companies often have. In the disaster recovery *business*, she argues, "needs are not met or eliminated faster," but more money is spent and much profit is made, usually by outsiders (174, 175; Adams 2012). Similar trends might be tracked in the world of global health.

Government resources in Sierra Leone have been cut back and expensive consultants are regularly flown in to "solve" local problems, at a cost far exceeding the use of local expertise. The problem of relying on foreign experts in efforts to solve global health problems is not new. For many years medical anthropologists have questioned the logic of using teams of World Health Organization experts over experts who know a good deal about how health is achieved, or not, in the places where aid is delivered. What is new, however, is how the metrics of global health get used to justify new kinds of experts—that is, those who know the metrics and how to produce them. On my flight to Freetown in 2014, I met one of these experts, who knew a good deal about how to calculate investment returns for the fund that wanted to build a hydroelectric dam but knew virtually nothing about the history, politics, health impacts, or local concerns over this dam (which had interrupted its construction for many years). This is where the metrics and reality meet up: statistical metrics and market logics can bypass local realities altogether and still meet investor expectations. Experts like this are able to make metrics do the challenging work of generating value and return, long before (and even without) knowing much about what happens on the ground in these communities. Many of the new global health and development metrics further authorize an "investors take all" sensibility in the global health work they do; how this all plays out on the ground is usually an afterthought.

Rich Is Different

There are fundamental differences in how people understand the financial instruments and arrangements of global health today; funding and investments are increasingly conflated in global health discourse, but they are not the same. Funding, from any source, produces expectations of intervention in relation to health outcomes, and this could be as banal and fundamental as making primary health care available in a new place. For many years governments invested in their own and other countries' health with just this sort of intention and ambition. Treating health as a financial investment, however, inevitably produces different expectations of return. Big investments produce expectations of big return, and in the process health and financial returns can become unself-consciously conflated. Investors expect to make money, whether they are governments, small do-good groups, or wealthy individuals. Investments are social mechanisms able to create demands and pressures on the development of global health technologies — not necessarily because they work to actually improve health but rather because they can make money. Shifting the model for financing health to the market shifts basic outcomes metrics from "Are you feeling better?" to "Did they make money?" As I have argued, the two don't necessarily overlap, despite the assumptions and rhetoric at places like the GHIF and BIO.

One of the most serious threats posed by new global health financial instruments and arrangements is the way they change our understanding of "care," shifting attention away from people's suffering to metrics that assume that if money has been made, some sort of care has been delivered. "The business of business is business," Friedman (1970) notes, and as I have previously found in the research of corporate managers and executives in Germany, actual health experiences often get obscured in the calculations used to determine success (Erikson 2012).

Many people have long assumed that challenges of global health would be remedied with more money. But putting more money into the system is not turning out to be the nostrum so many assumed. There is more money than ever before in human history going into human health, but even in many countries in the Organization for Economic Cooperation and Development we have begun to see downturns in public health gains in life expectancy and the management of metabolic syndrome (Swinburn et al. 2011). Some scholars have attributed this fact to the increasing influence of corporations and philanthropists in public health venues like the World Health Organization, where they regularly sit at the decision-making tables as "partners in health" (Lee et al. 2012), influencing decisions that are not actually in the best interest of population health but that do make money for powerful investors.

In fact having more and more corporate types (from JPMorgan to BIO) involved in the work of global health may point to one of the most significant health risks posed by commercial ventures: when the numbers go down, capital ventures leave. That is "business as usual." This is potentially a problematic model for sustainable health care systems; human health requires constancy over time and space and sometimes an ability to make decisions that are not solely based on fiscal concerns.

Conversations about what to do about wealth inequities have begun in earnest (see Piketty 2014), though it is too early to tell if there will be a lasting impact on contemporary logics about what will "fix" global health. We are moving more deeply into a world order where clinical and public health efforts are comingled with investment logics, and they do so through metrics. As a global community, we have not been nearly self-conscious or critical enough about what these new arrangements may mean for human health. A global health field driven by investors' expectations of return is a public health risk of yet unknown magnitude and scope.

Notes

1. In the United States from 2009 to 2012 the "top wealthiest 1% people's incomes grew by 31.4% while the remaining 99% incomes grew only by 0.4%" (Saez 2013).

2. The video link has been removed, but I watched and took notes from the video of panel presentations in 2011.

3. See http://ghif.com.

4. Susanne Craig, 2013. "Goldman Sachs, Buying Redemption," *New York Times*, October 26.

5. Reed Abelson, 2000. "Charities' Investing: Left Hand, Meet Right," *New York Times*, June 11.

6. Charles Piller, Edmund Sanders, and Robyn Dixon. 2007. "Dark Cloud over Good Works of Gates Foundation," *Los Angeles Times*, January 7.

7. Amy Goodman, 2007. "Gates Foundation Causing Harm with the Same Money It Uses to Do Good." *DemocracyNow!*, January 9. Accessed June 15, 2014. http://www .democracynow.org/2007/1/9/report_gates_foundation_causing_harm_with.

7 · WHEN GOOD WORKS COUNT LILY WALKOVER

Hesperian Health Guides' landmark publication, *Where There Is No Doctor,* is the most widely used primary health care book in the world, according to the World Health Organization. But the impact of the book is hard to quantify. It's hard to count numbers of copies used and numbers of lives saved when the intention of the book is to reach those without access to the formal health care system—people who, by definition, are hard to count. Still, philanthropy-funded global health institutions today are being asked to do just this: not just to count, but to count in specific ways that show, statistically, that things are working. As Sarah Shannon, the executive director of Hesperian, puts it, "'Can't you just send some books to one village, not to another, and then measure the difference?" At least ten potential funders have asked me that question. There's so much pressure to show fast, biometric impact, a sort of hegemony of biometrics, when what we do is capacity building. What we want to do at this point is to find a way to appropriately measure and document human capacity in a global health world dominated by the randomized controlled trial. The RCT is a one-size-fits-all model, and it doesn't leave space for long-term change, which is what we support. We may need funding, but we also want to protect the integrity of our work" (interview from field notes, January 28, 2014).

This chapter explores how humanitarianism takes up and is restructured by the demand for metrics in the context of global health. Taking into account the complex ways numbers and stories are grafted together to create narratives of deserving sufferers and capable donors, I explore the concept of "measurement," an idea based on the power of numbers, but more complex than numbers alone. I also explore models of resistance, including efforts to think about measurement and evaluation in ways that are built on an understanding of inherently messy social conditions and nuanced ideas of accountability. There are many domains within global health, and this paper focuses on the mid- or meso-level activities that emerge from institutions—specifically the global health nonprofit, or nongovernmental organization.

Often international in reach and communication but local in impact, these meso-level, ten- to fifty-person organizations are governed by boards of directors that frequently have liberal aims at heart and in many cases are openly critical of the large bureaucratic and conventional health development organizations that have typically been associated with large-scale numerical data production. I will demonstrate how, in using donor money and support to mitigate suffering in the lives of individuals—and to meet the accountability metrics those donors ask for—these NGOs become implicated in sustaining the very systems they criticize. If the "NGO-ization" of global health, a process Arundhati Roy (2011) describes as the rise of private-sector nonprofits to perform services previously supported by the public sector, is conditioned by both social movements and the economic pressures of neoliberal development policies, this new emphasis on metrics makes clear the contradictory position nonprofits fill in their capacity as organizations that are both created by a neoliberal economics of inequality (and the gaps left open by an underfunded state) and dependent upon funding from its ever-increasing fortunes.

Materials for this analysis are drawn from my experiences working at Hesperian Health Guides, a nonprofit public health publisher based in Berkeley, California, over a five-year period. Through an open copyright, Hesperian titles, including *Where There Is No Doctor*, have been translated into over eighty languages and used in 221 countries and territories (Hesperian Health Guides 2013). As an employee, I also attended numerous conferences and participated in global networks of nonprofits and health activists. In fall 2013 I conducted a pilot study that included interviews with individuals who have been involved in using, reviewing, and translating Hesperian materials. All the participants are doctors and established public health professionals working in different countries across sub-Saharan Africa, South Asia, and North and Central America, and many work with or run their own nonprofits. I also conducted fieldwork at the Hesperian offices and interviewed staff. My analysis is aimed at conveying a sense of how Hesperian and its partners work to make sense of the new types of demands that arrive in the form of a new metrics of accountability and to shed light on how these demands change the global health work that gets done in communities around the world.

Accounting for Global Health Humanitarianism

The story of how metrics became important to the work of Hesperian is in part the story of how humanitarian work became part of global health. Tracing the rise of humanitarianism in relation to the rise of global health offers an interesting set of insights about the intersection of the two as they have been structured by both the development paradigm and the post-colonial power dynamics that that paradigm set in motion. Specifically this history raises questions about who NGOs, as an institutional form, are accountable to, as well as how people and politics become both visible and invisible in this accountability. Hesperian's position in this intersection, and the organization's concepts of accountability — and countability — conflict with demands created by the structure of global health humanitarianism.

Humanitarianism has a long and complex history and has been explored in relation to the social factors that have most influenced it, including militarism (Chandler 2001), capitalism (Haskell 1985), and crisis (Fassin 2012; Rees forthcoming). Rees argues that humanitarianism is a relatively recent concept. The word itself was first used in English in 1838 to describe responses to the poverty created in the wake of the Industrial Revolution. This early humanitarianism distinguished itself from previous forms of religious charity through its focus on *society* as a field of intervention rather than the *individual*. It was, ironically, a type of "dehumanization" that created the concept of humanitarianism that we use today, and this dehumanization provided a new opportunity for intervention; from colonial subjects to slums of factory workers in Europe, there were whole societies waiting to be saved. Contemporary humanitarianism, or 'the humanitarian crisis,' first became possible in 1969, during "the first exclusively NGO run and organized large-scale humanitarian operation," organized in response to the Nigerian Civil War (Rees forthcoming: 12; see also Chandler 2001; De Waal 1997). As Rees notes, the rebel Ibo government of Biafra hired Markpress, a British public relations company, to share their plight with the world. As Markpress flooded the world with images of suffering Nigerians, "a few humanitarian organizations decided to ignore the principle of sovereignty. At stake was not the legal reaction of a nation—but humanity" (Rees forthcoming: 13). At the same time that other African countries were still fighting for independence from their colonizers, humanitarian organizations made their first postcolonial entrance into the continent, establishing the claim that the deserving sufferers they set out to help were part of a *global* humanity that came into visibility somewhere above and beyond the nation-state.[1]

The concurrent rise of late twentieth-century global health and development as a set of institutional commitments makes it clear that the politicization of humanitarian work is part of its *reason for being* even while it must transcend the politics of nation-states. The development of the World Health Organization in 1948 called attention to the need to respond to a global humanity that erased nation-state politics. *International health* "referred primarily to a focus on the control of epidemics between nations," while the newer term *global health* "implies consideration of the health needs of the people of the whole planet above the concerns of particular nations" (Brown et al. 2006: 62).[2]

This idea that the needs of people transcend the boundaries drawn by states—often as an excuse for the powerful to travel across those lines—is a recurring theme throughout the history of humanitarianism; the shift from *international* to *global* health reflects the same shift that emerged with the rise of the humanitarian crisis. This intersection emerged in the context of the development era, which Ananya Roy (2012) argues has been reformed over the past several decades around the global imaginary of poverty. The moral vision this imaginary invokes undergirds the global health humanitarianism that links humanitarian interventions to the new global antipoverty development paradigm. Roy argues that this formation "must be understood today as a global form of governing, one that exceeds both the state and the market" (107). The humanity it constructs can be intervened on regardless of state lines, while global health humanitarianism's enactment through tax-free charitable gifts and nonprofit organizations reinforces its place outside any one nation's political economy, but not beyond the global market.

Over time global health, emerging from international health enterprises, has expanded its vested interests in *knowing how others should live and teaching them about this* to *translating health and humanitarian needs into aid activities that can produce numerical results*.[3] These interests enabled certain claims to power, Tania Murray Li (2007) argues, often operating through a process she calls "rendering technical," a process that "confirms expertise and constitutes the boundary between those who are positioned as trustees, with the capacity to diagnose deficiencies in others, and those who are subject to expert direction" (7). In global health humanitarianism this process is increasingly dominated by requirements linking the production of metrics to financial support; trustees now determine the types of measurements necessary to document both the existence of the deserving poor and the progress they must show to remain deserving of intervention.

Hesperian Health Guides

The history of the rise of global health humanitarianism provides a useful backdrop to the history of the founding of Hesperian. As a legal entity Hesperian was first formed as a foundation to support the Biafra refugee crisis in the ferment of the San Francisco Bay Area's history of social activism and interest in liberation movements in the United States and abroad.[4] This social context also contributed to the travels of the founders that planted the seeds for how Hesperian would be transformed. Hesperian as it exists today originated with a group of volunteers led by a high school teacher from northern California who started working with village health workers after visiting the rural mountain town of Ajoya in Mexico.

Over time the group built up a small nonprofit organization that integrated the work of local community health workers and American volunteers to provide primary health care services to the town and to create short written materials on general health, training health workers, and supporting disabled village children. As these materials were being combined to form the book that would later be published as *Donde No Hay Doctor* in 1973 and translated into English as *Where There Is No Doctor* in 1977, the group needed nonprofit status in the United States to manage its finances.

It took over the charter of the Hesperian Foundation, whose work was ending as the civil war in Biafra died down.

As the idea of humanitarian crises was being solidified and a transnational intervene-able humanity created, Hesperian's mission shifted toward the idea that individuals have the capacity and knowledge to take care of themselves and their communities, inspired by the movement that grew out of Paulo Freire's (1970) popular education methodologies and was codified in the Alma Ata Declaration in 1978. Hesperian contested the depoliticized nature of the ethos of the humanitarian crisis, as well as the idea that outside intervention was the answer.

In the forty years since the publication of the first edition of *Where There Is No Doctor*, Hesperian has published nine additional books, and it has developed a participatory development process that institutionalizes the value of lay and community-based knowledge for health. Key to this process is field testing. When creating new material, Hesperian starts with a draft based on research conducted by staff and partners, carefully edited to be easy to read and use. The draft material is laid out with illustrations and sent out for different types of review. Medical reviewers provide feedback on diagnosis and treatment instructions; usually these are licensed medical professionals working in a variety of settings around the world. Field reviewers provide feedback on medical content and the overall presentation of material, based on their experiences working with communities that have limited access to the formal health system. Field testing is designed to directly elicit feedback from community members who will, ideally, use these books once they are published and translated.

Hesperian provides a small amount of funding to partner organizations to gather groups of their constituents—women in an HIV support group in South Africa, for example, or school children in Nepal—to share draft material and elicit feedback. The partners who conduct field testing often translate the material as they are testing it and read content out loud for participants who do not read or write. They discuss individual and group reactions and write up feedback to send back to Hesperian. When all three types of feedback have been collected, they are collated, and a team of editors plans what is usually a significant revision of the material. In this process field testing is valued equally with the medical and field review, based on the assumption that it is as important that the material be usable and useful to the intended audience as that it be technically accurate.

The invitation to cocreate Hesperian materials in some ways becomes even more significant after the initial publication of the books. Because the books are produced using an open copyright, partner organizations are invited to translate and adapt materials, and NGOs that conducted field testing are often the first to take up this next stage of the work. Through these networks Hesperian books travel, taking on different forms, but are usually recognizable by their line drawings (often redrawn for different contexts so that people can imagine themselves in the books), simple language, and titles. Translations also occur outside Hesperian's network, like the case of a Dari edition of *Where Women Have No Doctor* for Afghanistan, which Hesperian wasn't aware of until ten years after its publication, when the translators wrote to Hesperian to find out more about the organization. For Hesperian this global uptake is the real measure of success. If the books are useful to individuals and communities around the world, if they allow people to take action for their own health, then they have made an impact.

Contested Accountabilities: How Many Babies Did You Save Today?

Initially in the world of humanitarian aid, what was needed were lists of lives saved, pictures of mothers with their sweet-faced (formerly emaciated) children. Today money demands numbers. Now it is the randomized controlled trial, the RCT, that is used as the arbiter of value and worthiness (Adams 2013a; Erikson 2012). If a global health nonprofit can present its work as research-based, that's great; if it can present its work as a research intervention, that's even better. The revival of the idea that scientific methods can be used to better know and understand the messy morass of humanity has carefully distanced itself from memories of debunked colonial sciences such as craniometry (Gould 1996). Today science appears as an instrument of humanitarian aid. In all the major humanitarian foundations there is a growing emphasis on the production of numbers, and these show up in global health conferences around the world (Crane 2013).[5]

Today global health is globalizing science, and communities from big-city slums to small mountain towns are reimagined as extensions of clinical laboratories. "With effort, it was felt that they could be made to approximate . . . research spaces, conceptually and epistemologically" (Adams 2013a: 64; this volume). As "the field" became an extension of "the laboratory," work that had previously been judged primarily on outcomes specific to the location and situation have become sites of ambivalent value because of this specificity. They are now seen as worthy of funding and support only when able to generate statistical information that can be comparable across time and global geographic reaches.

Hales (this volume) builds on this critique, using the experiences of a Native Alaskan mental health program to explore the ways in which producing a supposedly universal "evidence-based evaluation" comes at a cost to valuing locally produced knowledge. She goes on to describe the cultural basis of metrical knowledge and how it contrasts with native Yup'ik formulations of knowledge. What is produced in the field of global health by prioritizing these types of culturally specific scientific questions? First, a simplification of complex social dynamics down to numbers, and second, a contested field in which different players—including those being counted—work to shape and negotiate the evaluations that will define how and where money is allocated.

As a U.S.-based nonprofit organization, Hesperian relies on a combination of grants from foundations, gifts from individual donors, and book sales. Donors have always asked for accountability, to know that their dollars are going toward good work. However, in the past decade there has been a significant rise in requests for a certain kind of measurement of that good work. This has been matched by a request for specificity and a short timeframe. For example, one funder who was approached for what would become Hesperian's *A Community Guide to Environmental Health* was interested in funding the development of material about only one particular kind of toilet. Not only would they not consider funding the full section on sanitation (which includes instructions on how to build seven different types of toilets, depending on community needs, resources, and the local environment), but they wanted to know specifically how many fewer children would die of diarrhea and dehydration in Tanzania in the three years after they provided the funding.

Hesperian did its best to show a causal link and provide an estimated number. However, the value of the information about toilets was complemented by information on oral rehydration salts, water purification methods and techniques for reducing standing water during the rainy season. With a comprehensive approach, it isn't possible to point to one intervention that made a change—and in many cases it isn't desirable. In some communities knowing how to build that one new type of toilet may have really made a difference. In others the introduction of a new water purification technique or the realization that oral rehydration solution can be made at home rather than purchased at a pharmacy might have made the difference.

These demands for measurement—especially when trying to measure human capacity over time—also put pressure on staff time and impact the kind of work that gets done. Administering different funding sources that individually cover only a small piece of work—and require people and deficits to be counted—takes up valuable time.

Another experience at Hesperian provides an example of this. In an effort to produce a statistical accounting of their success in order to meet donor expectations, Hesperian fundraisers felt pressured to include a before-and-after survey to measure whether the field-testing process was "empowering" to the participants in a grant. Some staff tasked with carrying out the survey, however, believed that such tactics would imply that the target community could be characterized by what it was missing and the degree to which it had attained a goal set by Hesperian. This constituted an infringement on the methods the organization used to elicit participation and empowerment; in fact, they argued, it would potentially undermine these goals. The staff felt that the survey was asking the partners, generally grassroots groups doing community work and very busy, to spend valuable time on measuring their own supposed lack of empowerment. This was a conflict in terms of time spent, and staff feared it might be insulting to the partners.

In the end the survey was carried out to satisfy the funder, and a significant amount of time that would have otherwise gone toward the development of the book and the running of the field test partner's programs was devoted instead to developing and completing the survey. Although concerns about the survey and its utility were expressed, the same survey format appeared in a grant for a different book project a few years later, under similar pressure. As Biruk (2012) notes, the mandate to craft interventions as research projects permeates the most remote global sites as part of the global health nonprofit world. In order to see like a research project, NGOs today are asked to transform social reality into problems that can be fixed and funded, and managing uncertainties inherent in human behavior and interaction becomes inextricably tied to processes of data production. In carrying out a survey to evaluate an established practice that in some ways undermined the practice itself—requesting that partners who are being asked to contribute their expertise on health content first report on their lack of empowerment—Hesperian acquiesced to pressure to *count deficits* in order to justify funding.

Internally Hesperian sees itself as ultimately accountable to the users of its books: community health workers, community organizers, and anyone without access to health care and the resources necessary for health. Externally, however, Hesperian and many other nonprofit organizations like it are dependent on donor foundations, and those donors often see accountability through the promissory lenses and rubrics being offered by metrics as a new evidence base. Foundations generally see organizations as accountable to them for the money they have provided rather than both the foundation and the organization being accountable to the community they hope to work with and serve. In global health, donors want to measure this accountability in numbers, and often more specifically in biometrics—specific health outcomes with direct causal links to health interventions. Of course real community health comes about through complex interactions and multiple causal pathways. A healthy environment, strong community ties, and sustainable infrastructure for health care cannot be delivered by "intervention"; they must be built up over time by community participation and local ownership—a message Freire was committed to.

Looking for New Models

From Hesperian's perspective, there are three main issues with the current metrics-driven funding and accountability models in global health humanitarianism, each of which can be pushed back against in different ways. The first is that it is very difficult to measure and document human capacity. The rise and dominance of the RCT in global health and development work makes it hard to justify other ways of understanding individual and community growth and change to funders, but there are efforts to do just that being developed by researchers, organizations, and in some cases funders themselves. Outcome mapping, which emphasizes change over time and recognizes the agency of people making change in their own communities, is one such methodology that Hesperian is experimenting with. Outcome mapping is a method of tracking a project that is based on the idea that people make change in their own communities and that funding organization should not expect to be able to measure a direct impact; instead they will be able to see the effect of their work on intermediaries, who then make the direct change in their own communities (Mertens and Wilson 2012; Outcome Mapping Learning Community n.d.). It is an ongoing and cyclical methodology, which involves tracking change over time, assuming that capacity building takes time and functions through ongoing relationships.

The second issue that Hesperian runs up against is the timeframe: funders want short-term measurable results and often are not willing to support or wait for long-term impact. Once again this makes it difficult to observe social change and human capacity building. One of the indicators of social change that Hesperian is looking for in its outcome mapping project is a person being inspired by his or her use of the books to become a health worker or health activist. But counting inspiration is not only difficult conceptually; it also takes time away from other kinds of health education work. The kind of shift in personal goals they are being asked to quantify usually takes place organically over years, starting with, for example, a person who comes across a copy of *Where There Is No Doctor* and uses it to take care of his or her own health or the health of someone in the family. Next that person might use the book to give advice to a neighbor, and over time more people come to ask for advice. In some cases that person is inspired to start a community-based organization, in others to go and get formal training so that he or she can continue to support the health of the community directly. Again, making all of this information speak in numbers is time-consuming and costly.

The third issue that Hesperian is attempting to address is the fact that the metrics organizations are asked to produce are usually determined by funders without grassroots input. This goes against the working model of the organization, which tries to do its work from the bottom up, following an anticolonialist and anti-imperialist Freirean philosophy that starts from the assumption that all people have the ability to think critically and are the best positioned to understand their own needs and resources. The metrics demands of funders, despite their often good intentions to ensure that only "effective" work is done, come from an imperialist frame that assumes those at the top of the power structure have the clearest view of the needs, resources, and abilities of those below. Added to this challenge is the fact that there is sub rosa pressure to report only positive findings. Again this goes against the organization's ethos of learning from the community and adapting to specific community contexts. Without room to fail, Hesperian staff argue, the field isn't able to learn from its own mistakes or to remain accountable to the local populations it serves.

As the trustees of global health ask for more numbers, they are reshaping the kinds of work that nonprofits do and the kinds of services and resources that are provided to communities. People at every level—community members and organizers, nonprofits functioning in the field of the Global South and the office of the Global North, and even the staff of the funding organizations themselves—spend more and more time making the world into a place that can be calculated more precisely in order to be intervened in. Despite the sincere aspirations of those who use these scientific methods to improve the lives of suffering people, it is worth asking where these aspirations are undermined by the fact that only knowledge produced within the discursive terms of these narrow metrics is counted as valid. How does this process elide and efface other kinds of evidence and other kinds of knowledge that are critical to effective global health outcomes? When does this process take crucial time and resources away from the very social programs it hopes to make possible?

Partnership and Valuable Inequalities

Global health humanitarianism is based on what Johanna Crane (2013) calls "valuable inequalities." Poverty creates opportunities for those with concentrated wealth to intervene in the lives of others and to create data and tell stories to document and justify their interventions. All of this can be for the good; that is, such an alliance is not inherently unfair or problematic. Still Crane identifies the development of global health at the "productive but troubling nexus between disaster, assistance, and scientific opportunity" (7) as a nexus we should be careful about. For meso-level global health nonprofits, that nexus intersects with the existence of jobs and organizations that are trying to, and often succeeding in, doing a lot of good work.

NGOs like Hesperian offer an important complement to government and bilateral or multilateral work and to large international NGOs that are defining how to do global health today. Hesperian is part of a generation of nonprofits developed during the primary health care movement and Alma Ata, focused on self-determination, the right to health, and the idea that technical information can be taken up by anyone (as opposed to the current trend, which assumes that technical information should be used to create tools that can be used to intervene on anyone).

Today the relationships and partnerships between rights-based NGOs and large government and multilateral organizations are such that the former are being asked to incorporate practices of quantification that may or may not help them achieve their goals, a request that trickles down from donor infrastructures that request a specific kind of accountability. In turn these pressures help form the basis of new organizations, which often incorporate gathering metrics on an equal footing with their other goals. This new aspect of unequal global health partnerships—agreeing to be measured and helping to measure oneself, as Hesperian's partners did for the field test empowerment survey and as scores of organizations ask of their recipients—deserves some skepticism.

Hesperian's model of partnership—in which field partners are assumed to be the more knowledgeable of the two—is one potential model that could be proposed as a counterpoint to some sort of metrics and some sort of accountability. While there will always be pressure for measurement in some form as justification for funding, Hesperian's demonstrates that the underlying assumption that there are different kinds of knowledge and different ways of measuring (many of which do not originate in the scientific labs of the Global North) needs to be kept in mind.

The rise of global health metrics both reinforces and reshapes global health humanitarianism by requiring particular kinds of measurement of efforts that range from direct service provision to community organizing. How these metrics become instruments of what Adams defines as a new kind of 'global sovereign' in the first chapter of this volume—"a flexible assemblage of data production" that "orchestrates biopolitical health interventions so that they work within capitalism's terms and limits"—is very much tied up in questions of what kind of knowledge those metrics employ to determine accountability and efficacy.

As global health trustees reach across borders and intervene in the lives of whole groups of people and in the structure of health aid as it is implemented by governments, multilateral bodies, and nonprofits, these questions of metrics become all the more important. If we adopt the idea that only those who can be counted can (or should) be seen as deserving (of partnership or intervention, depending on the model of work), we run the risk of erasing many of the people we most want to include in our work. RCT methods in particular often ignore root causes of health problems, and they run the risk of validating short-term, vertical solutions that don't question the way that politics of resource extraction and distribution create and exacerbate inequality in the first place.

In Defense of Good Work

Accountability, as a concept, is important for the development of strong, productive relationships that emerge in efforts to improve the health of communities around the world. New kinds of alliances with funders who are interested in supporting more nuanced, qualitative, and long-term capacity building and social change are key, and a number of funders are beginning to understand this. The desire — in many religions and cultures, the *command* — to help those in need is a noble endeavor, but it is also an intrinsically complicated one. Unequal power dynamics that come with helping the poor often give the donor a kind of power that is undeserved, and even undesired. However, this only calls all the more urgently on those of us working in this field to resist the pull of what seems to be neat and clean, fast and simple problem solving through metrics and to instead think long and hard about how we think of numbers, what kinds of metrics we really need, and what kinds of outcomes we really want. Global health metrics, implemented through humanitarian means, promise a lot — better medicines, healthier people — and they produce valuable information and solutions. But when they are assumed to be more valuable than the knowledge that people have about their own lives and conditions, they obscure something much more important.

Notes

1. For this analysis I am distinguishing these "humanitarian" groups from other philanthropies that were involved with international health work, tropical medicine, and colonial regimes (Rockefeller Foundation, Ford Foundation, etc.) at the time.

2. In this history they also trace the brief prominence of primary health care in the 1960s and 1970s as the World Health Organization's push for comprehensive primary health care and health for all by the year 2000 was replaced by a neoliberal metrics-driven "selective" primary health care campaign. *Where There Is No Doctor* was an important part of the grassroots movement that created the energy for the World Health Organization's brief primary health care push. As a member of the People's Health Movement, Hesperian has also critiqued vertical health programming and pushed for a revitalization of comprehensive primary health care at a policy level.

3. To further understand the type of governance that is being implicated in this sce-

nario, I turn to Murray Li's (2007) exploration of improvement schemes in Indonesia. She lays out the idea of trusteeship, "a position defined by the claim to know how others should live, to know what is best for them, to know what they need" (4).

4. The Hesperian Foundation was named after the street that the organization's first offices were on. In 2011 Hesperian legally changed its name to Hesperian Health Guides in order to more accurately reflect the organization's mission.

5. Of course there have been objections to this narrowed definition of global health knowledge by grassroots groups and health activists around the world, and the foundations and conference organizers have made some accommodations. "Civil society" is now consulted, invited to contribute to panels and reports, or at least to provide commentary. Civil society, however, is often composed of nonprofit professionals whose experience of the "community's" struggles is negotiated through their own position as a crossover subject, an expert representative of the poor and disenfranchised.

PART IV. STORIED METRICS

8 · WHEN NUMBERS AND STORIES COLLIDE Randomized Controlled Trials and the Search for Ethnographic Fidelity in the Veterans Administration CAROLYN SMITH-MORRIS

Assuming both are medically stable, a fifty-three-year-old American computer programmer with tetraplegia from an injury sustained in fighting in Vietnam typically has a lot more job options than a recently injured American thirty-eight-year-old roofer with the same SCI. But they look about the same in randomized controlled trial (RCT) data. Why? Because, in the stripped-down language of clinical trials, facts about people are homogenized in order to foster clear outcomes in relation to a small set of isolated factors. The U.S. medical system's reliance on these unembellished metrics and the austere research designs that support them has far-reaching implications not only for health (especially for persons with SCI) but for entire health care infrastructures. Here, at what some might call the center and others might call the periphery of the global health community, we find trends in the use of metrics that are simultaneously specific and global in significance.

Drawing from research within the largest integrated health care system in the United States, the Veterans Health Administration (VHA), I examine some of the challenges of bringing qualitative data and research methodologies to bear within the politically charged, outcome-driven context of a U.S. government institution. My experience as a researcher in one RCT among veterans with spinal cord injury serves as a case study for this chapter. Increasingly all forms of care and all types of healers and care providers are pressed by market-driven biomedical ideologies to funnel all outcomes evidence into the RCT mold. The state colludes with this pressure through organizations like the VHA and asserts new levels of conformity in both patient and professional populations. But using these models to decipher outcomes and determine optimal modes of care can be misleading, sometimes promoting metric quantification over case-specific quality, which, after all, is the ultimate outcome of care. I will document a project that illustrates how both the work of the RCT and the kinds of information that the RCT fails to acknowledge reveal and create gaps even while trying to ensure that these disparate metrics are integrated. I wish to show how numbers and stories can be used collaboratively but also in ways that are fraught in large institutions of health care. The VHA, which meets the needs and rights of U.S. veterans for not only health care but for the best that scientific research can supply, exposes the collision of numeracy and ethnographic data in global health metrics.

The Quality Revolution(s)

At the beginning of my career in the late 1980s, hospital care was monitored through systems of quality assurance, or what was also called quality *improvement* (based on the hyperproductive and efficient Japanese companies from which the Deming model and team concepts emerged). Quality monitoring, then and now, includes everything from reducing errors in medical record transcription and drug delivery to utilization review (nurses with insurance or actuarial expertise) and having agreements in place for the transportation of psychotic patients by bus, using physical and chemical restraints if necessary. One of my first positions was assisting, and eventually leading, the Quality Improvement Office and accreditation review cycles of a mental health hospital. So my sensitivity to this language of quality, measurement, monitoring, and evidence has been long in the making.

By the 1990s "quality" health care was infused with customer service messaging, lessons in "total quality management," and the need to foster cultures of "continuous quality improvement" so that every worker and every patient was empowered to identify, and then act, to correct or improve upon a problem (Lammers et al. 1996).[1] My position was an irritant to many of the hospital staff and a necessary evil in the world of increasingly "managed" and "accredited" health care that had to be done in ways that demonstrated both good quality and a continuous effort to measure and improve.

The early 1990s was also a time during which the VHA—the national health system designed for research, health care, and health insurance for the honorably discharged veterans of the U.S. armed forces—had a reputation for *poor* quality care (Oliver 2007). In the era of total quality management and continuous quality improvement, the VHA was under tremendous pressure to transform itself using Deming models or any other means necessary. The secretary of the VHA at the time was widely hailed as revolutionary. His campaigns included a major reorganization of the lines of authority and decision making across this vast system, increased emphasis on primary care over inpatient and acute care, implementation of an electronic health record, and the development of "a larger sustained effort to systematically study and enhance VHA clinical programs, including their quality, processes, and outcomes" (McQueen et al. 2004: 340).[2] Part of this transformation was QUERI, the VHA Quality Enhancement Research Initiative,[3] so by the mid-1990s the era of "quality" at the VHA had begun. Over the next decade there was tremendous growth in the QUERI program, and by the late 2000s quality in VHA care was reported by some to have been not only completely transformed but better than private care available in the United States (Kizer et al. 2008; Kupersmith et al. 2007; Oliver 2007; Stetler et al. 2008). Even so, yet another swing of the pendulum would bring wait times, limited prescription benefits, and hospital error to the Veterans Administration (VA) system, and to the news media as well. In 2009 the appointment of a new secretary of the VA was intended to produce another necessary massive transformation in addressing quality of care problems (Demakis et al. 2000; Kizer et al. 2008; McQueen et al. 2004), and this led to sixteen key initiatives, seven of which explicitly targeted the VHA and health benefits. The 2014 media frenzy over wait times and other "quality" issues (e.g., veteran homelessness, poor quality mental health care) led to this secretary's resignation. McCullough et al. (2013: 10) wrote prophetically, "VA leadership . . . [is] under public scrutiny and any adverse event could trigger ripples of political consequences that could potentially go all the way up to Capitol Hill." These types of political drama, in which heads of organizations take the fall for the most egregious—or most public— errors, is neither new nor noteworthy. But the relevance of this particular history for the VA, and specifically for the VHA and its dual treatment- research role in the nation's largest health care system, is disquieting.

The new national (and global) obsession with accountability for quality health care—for veterans through the VHA, for the uninsured through the Affordable Care Act, or "Health for All" through the World Health Organi- zation—suggests how performance metrics, outcome quantification, and the quantification of quality have been drawn deeply into the global public consciousness. In the United States responsibility for these practices fell squarely on the government. The past twenty years of VHA history are a microcosm in the progression of quality metrics and the types of evidence- based medicine that have been promoted through private and public sec- tor health policies. The continuing cycles of quality decline, followed by heroic and revolutionary change, play back like repeating cycles in a day- time television drama. One wonders whether the same volatility is evident at the granular and local level and whether the contentious marriage of state policy with market-driven cost-effective health care and medical re- search outside of the VHA is equally volatile.

Producing Qualitative Data in a Clinical Trial

The VHA is staffed by thousands of clinical and health science researchers, 60 percent of whom are also clinicians. And there are at least twenty-five anthropologists in the VA (Gemmae Fix, personal communication, Janu- ary 8, 2015). As in other teaching hospitals, VHA research institutions are a blend of academic and clinical space, merging these two pursuits into complex and dynamic work relationships with varying degrees of success. Research is conducted for multiple reasons in the VHA, but the most pub- lic of these reasons is "to fulfill VHA's core research missions through a di- verse portfolio of medical (basic and clinical), rehabilitation, and health services research" (McQueen et al. 2004: 339). In its various websites, stra- tegic plans, and literature, the VHA takes pride in combining research with clinical care as a way to "identify the direct needs of patients at chair and bedside, and to find discoveries and innovations directly in-step with these needs—keeping the Veteran at the center of health care from the very beginning."[4]

The VHA manages research through its Office of Research and Development. The budget request for this vast national research program for 2015 was over $589 million.[5] The dual responsibilities of the VHA as provider of clinical care for a politically influential and highly symbolic segment of the population (i.e., to care for "him who shall have borne the battle and for his widow, and his orphan," according to Abraham Lincoln, who supplied the original motto of the VA) and as a competitive research center with direct ties to and corresponding obligations under federal funding, make the VHA an intriguing incubator for policy reverb, feedback on fiscal priorities, and scientific echo.[6]

The VHA trial for which I was hired as a contract medical anthropologist was designed to promote quality of life for veterans with spinal cord injury (SCI), one of ten focal areas for which a QUERI Coordinating Center was established. The project was integrally part of the VHA agenda for quality monitoring, research producing evidence of best practice, and the granting of research dollars through the VA system to specialized VHA sites across the nation. My role was to provide supplemental qualitative data about a trial that was already in full swing by the time I arrived. This role gave me insights on the quality and evidence-based medicine agenda within the trial and, more generally, on how these forces impact researchers who design and conduct trials.[7]

The project, called Spinal Cord Injury Vocational Integration Program: Implementations and Outcomes (SCI-VIP), was a multicenter clinical trial evaluating the impact of evidence-based supported employment for veterans with SCI. It was mostly organized around the performance of specific services and the collection of quantitative data on outcomes, but the purpose of the qualitative research (in which I was involved) was to describe the universe of experiences and opinions represented in the illness narratives of participants and staff. Research methods included semistructured and open-ended interviews with staff and participants, observations of provider-participant encounters, and participant observation in clinical and service activities as well as veterans' homes and communities. We also observed several staff meetings on a semiregular basis.[8] Ethnographic interviews with veterans occurred exclusively in community and home settings. In all interviews and conversations, key foci were (1) experiences of the veteran within the project or in the VA system of care generally, (2) the veteran's story of and perspective on the injury, (3) the meaning of work and the veteran's goals related to work, and (4) experiences and feelings about being a veteran and receiving care through the VHA. Not surprisingly these data were not being captured in the trial's original protocol.

Turning Support into a "Model"

Although my discussion in this chapter focuses on the outcome metrics of the trial, a brief introduction to the unique target of this trial is necessary. Were it not for an arguably extreme version of patient-centeredness in this model and the trial's commitment of fidelity to that model, I surely would not have two forms of evidence to discuss. As late as just one decade ago, patients recovering from SCI were discouraged from thinking about goals such as paid employment (Hammell 2007). Rehabilitation focused solely on physical rehabilitation, and critics noted that therapy was "treating the SCI but not the person who had sustained the SCI" (269). The Supported Employment model outlines an integrated approach to helping people obtain and maintain community-based competitive employment in their chosen occupations (Becker et al. 2006; Bond et al. 2001; Bond 2004). In the model a vocational rehabilitation counselor is seen as an integrated member of the existing interdisciplinary SCI team. The counselor is given more structured access to and is able to utilize and call upon the treatment team and its resources to enhance vocational rehabilitation services. This aspect of the model is not only distinctive and new but also crucial. That is, the counselor, rather than the patient, is now responsible for integrating and coordinating all vocational rehabilitation services, including job-finding efforts (which I describe later). In short the counselor is designed to serve a broader scope of duties in managing treatment for the patient and for collaborating with clinical and employment professionals.

One challenge of Supported Employment interventions was in creating an evidence base that would support its use. Evidence-based approaches had not been widely used or clinically tested among persons with physical disabilities, including SCI. Using the Supported Employment approach was already hard to accomplish and even harder to quantify. Unemployment for veterans with spinal injuries is a serious and common problem, contributing to lower reported quality of life, life satisfaction, and adjustment (Chapin and Kewman 2001; Krause 1990, 1992; Trieschmann 1980; Westgren and Levi 1998; Yerxa and Baum 1986), and our trial was meant to remedy precisely this set of problems. Thus one of the goals of the research was to find ways to acknowledge the veteran with SCI as a person in context, requiring coherence among the physical, emotional, and vocational aspects of his or her life. Still it was not entirely clear how to do an evidence-based version of RCT research that would provide data to show this.

The clinical researchers had to demonstrate the effectiveness of this program in ways the QUERI and the clinical and funding worlds would recognize. The research therefore adopted the gold standard trial methodology and the guidelines for reporting results of an RCT, including measures of *fidelity* to an evidence-based model of care, in this case supported employment. What these RCT efforts suggest is a rather large chasm between the qualitative data that make sense of these interventions and the quantitative requirements used in accounting for their outcomes.

Two Views of the Same Trial

Two of the RCT's published products reveal some of the tensions between the kinds of data QUERI needed (Ottomanelli, 2012, Effectiveness of Supported Employment for Veterans with spinal cord injuries: Results from a randomized multisite study). One (Ottomanelli et al. 2012) was written for a clinical journal conforming to RCT-driven models called the Consolidated Standards for Reporting Trials, or CONSORT. The original CONSORT statement (Begg et al. 1996; Moher et al. 2001) was written in 1996, with revisions in 2001 and 2010, to improve the quality of reporting so that readers of a published report would have access to "complete, clear, and transparent information on its methodologies and findings" (Schulz et al. 2010: 1). Using CONSORT was important because only certain forms and venues of publication (e.g., CONSORT publications for RCTs or PubMed-indexed journals) were (and are) valued within the VHA (McCullough et al. 2013).

The other published products were written for an anthropological journal and an edited volume (Smith-Morris et al. 2013, 2014). The differences between traditional RCT outcome data and traditional ethnographic data are great, but both studies were needed to adequately account for the trial's design, performance, and achievements. In the end the differences between these forms of evidence, or data, reveal some of the challenges in defining "quality" when it comes to outcomes, along with challenges involved in information gained or lost in this federally funded and government-affiliated research. My intention in making this contrast is not to disparage or applaud either perspective but rather to consider the spectacular voids cre-ated by CONSORT guidelines for RCT publication and the comparative messiness of the ethnographic accounts.

The CONSORT guidelines include a checklist of twenty-five items of in-formation to include when reporting an RCT. Among these are methods for randomization, allocation, and blinding; details on participant flow, re-cruitment, outcomes, and estimation; and discussion of limitations, gener-alizability, and interpretations (Schulz et al. 2010). Most PubMed-indexed journals require that authors follow these guidelines. In fact, however, it be-came quickly apparent that what the RCT CONSORT guidelines called for is *fidelity* and *outcome* statistics, not necessarily empirical or complete details about which aspects of the program worked and which did not.

Fidelity

The term *fidelity* refers to whether a trial's intervention was conducted con-sistently and completely as outlined in the model's protocol. Clinical trials that adopt the fidelity approach rigorously monitor, coach, and supervise the services performed to ensure ideal adherence to the intervention model (Bond et al. 2008a, 2008b). Values associated with the fidelity approach in-clude replicability of data and the reliability with which researchers can attest that the model, as designed, was indeed what occurred during re-search. Fidelity to the treatment model is considered one of the requisite metrics of scientific rigor in an RCT.[9] Fidelity was described in the clini-cal journal *Archives of Physical Medicine and Rehabilitation* this way: "The 3 [project] sites providing [Supported Employment] were evaluated every 6 months using the 15-item IPS Fidelity Scale. No differences in Fidelity scores over time or between sites in these biannual visits were observed during the study period ($F_{7, 18}$ = 0.8, $P<.619$; range, 59–68). A review of each site's fidelity ratings suggests significant achievement toward good [Supported Employment] implementation. As a whole, site fidelity scores averaged 63.4±2.5, which falls within the upper portion of the 'fair' range. Fidelity scores for staffing (12.8±0.5), organization (11.6±1.6), and services (38.9±1.5) demonstrated little change over the study period" (Ottomanelli et al. 2012: 743–44). In this reporting of fidelity scores, the emphasis is on how closely the intervention adhered to its procedural (and paperwork) protocols. But these numbers do not (and do not claim to) report the em-pirical outcomes of the intervention. In other words, even if the study had been conducted perfectly according to the model's protocols, the outcome could have been poor. Fidelity and outcome are not the same.

The quotation from Ottomanelli et al. (2012) reports an overall fidelity score for the model as a whole, then adds others for staffing, organization, and services rendered. Adhering to individual principles in the published supported employment model (e.g., measures of how well the vocational rehabilitation [VR] counselor was integrated into the clinical team or the degree to which care was multidisciplinary and how that actually worked) are *not*, however, part of this scoring system. Indeed fidelity metrics give only a broadly aggregated sense of how well the model was followed and which aspects of the model might have been more challenging.

The numbers claim fidelity as one success of the RCT; that is, the treatment model was implemented successfully, according to its terms and principles. However, these metrics offer very little "evidence" of any of the ethnographically significant findings relevant to the performance of the model. For instance, one principle of the model emerged over others in importance, and some principles required tremendous intensity of effort that was completely invisible in trial outcome or even fidelity metrics. The importance of these themes emerged only through analysis of the narrative accounts we gathered. Grounded analyses of multiple recorded and transcribed interviews with staff (with whom excellent rapport and trust had been developed over time) involved two independent rounds of coding of interview transcripts and analysis toward consensus of the relative importance of emergent themes—in other words, the *qualitative* research methodologies and the *qualitative* evidence. Still, for the CONSORT guidelines, the authors had to render this material legible as a metric of fidelity.

To be sure, fidelity monitoring helped the trial by ensuring that the principles were given appropriate attention and support during the trial. But the fidelity scores did *not* reveal the relative importance of things like integration or intensity of effort to the rest of the Supported Employment model's principles and to the trial's overall success in this site. Thus the fidelity report in clinical format, while affirming that the trial met this CONSORT requirement for trial evidence, is a limited data set.

Integration

The integration of the VR counselor into the clinical team's meetings, activities, and planning was itself somewhat revolutionary. A crucial and distinctive part of the Supported Employment model, integration envisions employment (historically an element of patients' lives that was considered part of their social context, and therefore largely irrelevant to clinical care) as part of all health care. VR counselor integration was discussed in the clinical publication this way: "Given the complexity of issues and barriers faced by individuals with SCI, there may be many reasons why [Supported Employment] has benefits for this population over conventional methods of VR. For one, this model involves integrating vocational services within the medical rehabilitation health care setting. This integration meant that the interdisciplinary health care team, which included the VR specialist, would identify and address barriers with the Veterans as they began a job search, as well as after the job was obtained and new issues emerged" (Ottomanelli et al. 2012: 746).

Given the inability of fidelity statistics to say much about how integration actually occurred, we do not learn how the VR counselor accomplished the very clear agenda laid out in the goals of the project. How, on the other hand, could it be shown that the VR counselor in the SCI-VIP did so much more than her non–Supported Employment counterparts? And how could all of these contextual barriers to positive outcomes become data points for reporting of outcomes? What I am drawing attention to is that even though the RCT reported fidelity, the very nuanced information about what made this intervention work better than previous models formed an evidence base that did not show up in these reports.

In contrast the ethnographic publications considered this process in detail. Things that were invisible in fidelity reporting became immediately obvious in the ethnographic research: a portion of the VR counselor's success was attributable to a smaller caseload; another portion to her longevity in similar work and familiarity with the local job markets; still another to her positive and constructive relationships with colleagues both in and outside of the trial—and even the VA—who shared cultural and social capital with her relevant to this work. However, as ethnographers learned when we duplicated the VR counselor's driving and home and employer visit schedule, the time savings of the smaller caseload were quickly and completely overrun by travel time to homes and communities within a hundred-mile radius of the office.

Ethnographers also watched and recorded as the VR counselor accessed and utilized the treatment team's resources, including clinical professionals and knowledge central to SCI rehabilitation. Persons with these injuries have more frequent medical complications, such as urinary tract infections, skin issues, or depression. The counselor communicated directly with the veterans' physicians, sped up medical attention when necessary, and offered input to treatment planning and healing that enabled quicker returns to work. The counselor also conducted job finding and utilized techniques like job carving, job coaching, and follow-along with employers to ensure the veterans' medical status met or exceeded their workplace demands.

As staff talked about the Supported Employment principles and the challenges of meeting these guidelines, integration of care (principle #1) was named far more often than any other as critical to their success.[10] At team meetings, we heard these sorts of comments: "[In the inpatient team meetings] we talk about cases—things that have happened with their medical [condition], things that have happened with people and how that has interfered or helped, how that impacted. . . . Or maybe good things, like so-and-so had a medical issue that came up and [the VR counselor] rapidly referred him to me and we took care of it and avoided a problem. . . . [The VR counselor] came to our [inpatient department] meeting [to tell us about this problem], and those are things that help." This staff member is describing a novel feature of the SCI-VIP: the counselor's regular access to the inpatient clinical team—the same team of clinicians who cared for the client when he or she first received the SCI. Research staff members augmented the importance of this sort of evidence by saying things like the following:

> When the [inpatient] staff meeting occurs, we try to give an update on [SCI-VIP] enrollment. . . . We try to kind of keep it in the forefront of [the clinical staff's] minds. We've been trying to kind of translate the success stories back to the team, so that they can see kind of the fruits of their labor in terms of what actually is happening and try to facilitate some of that mutual learning process between the vocational clinician and the SCI clinician that didn't previously have any exposure to what voc rehab meant. So, you know, the vocational clinician maybe doesn't know what an [occupational therapist] does and so we've been sort of trying to cultivate this cross, the integration.

Cultivating communication and mutual support between the VR counselor and the other experts on the clinical team is a key part of integration of care and is named by multiple types of staff as a key to the success of the Supported Employment model. By educating the clinical team on the principles and methods of the Supported Employment model, the trial expanded the normal purview of that team well beyond the clinic and into the communities and work settings of their patients. Likewise clinical integration of the counselor promoted her greater knowledge of and sensitivity to the medical needs of veterans, yielding greater success in her work.

Not surprisingly none of these kinds of data is available in the clinical publication. This is partly because so little room is available after CON-SORT requirements are met. Thus, despite the fact that my collaborating researchers *did* mention several of the ethnographic findings in the report, the standard reporting format dictated that the ethnographic detail be relegated to a different article and a different journal. In other words, the CON-SORT requirements did not account for what we considered to be the most important kinds of evidence for why the program worked. We do not see this as simply a problem of publication conventions. Rather it is a problem of what kinds of evidence count in the reporting of success and to whom these data count.

Intensity of Effort

Central to the purpose of the RCT was demonstration that the Supported Employment model of care was better than the traditional vocational rehabilitation model of care. That is, consistent with RCT designs, we used comparisons to establish impact effect. But a major factor in explaining the failure of the VR model was its generally lower likelihood of actually providing services (i.e., not that their actual services were less effective). The clinical publication had this to say: "It has been our observation that when Veterans are referred to providers or agencies outside the SCI center, relatively few of them actually receive any VR services. This is supported by our study finding that Veterans in the [Supported Employment] group had twice as many VR visits than those who were referred outside the SCI center for vocational care" (Ottomanelli et al. 2012: 746).

The Supported Employment model being tested addressed this problem (nonreceipt of services) explicitly. The model calls for "rapid engagement," "zero exclusion," and "ongoing support," making an exceptionally intensive job for the VR counselor. We saw similar trends in relation to what researchers called "intensity of effort": how much effort was put into support services for each veteran.

In the traditional model clients come to the VR counselor, but in the Supported Employment model VR involves numerous home visits and intensive support. One VR counselor, for example, had a client who lived at the near maximum distance of the catchment area (one hundred miles). The drives to see him were long, and his reluctance to visit with the counselor (even at his own home) was exacerbated by his drug use. In the traditional VR model, this man might never have received support for employment because those supports were available only in a professional office. The trial's VR counselor made this problem clear: "I had a guy in Fort Worth, who had an obvious drug problem and didn't want anyone in his house. He hated company. He admitted to me he signed on [to the SCI-VIP] just to get the fifty dollars [research stipend] every month. So I continued to go out there, you know. Then he started to get angry, because he didn't really want me to visit . . . but I continued to go out anyway. Just kept going, kept going, kept trying to talk to this guy. And he and I started to get along pretty well" (Smith-Morris et al. 2014: 148).

Through persistence and a flexible approach to goal setting, the VR counselor established rapport and was able to help this client get two job interviews prior to close of the trial, a much better result than traditional methods of VR might have achieved. The VR counselor reflected on the difficulty of achieving the same outcome (i.e., paid employment) with clients who start in such different states of readiness: "That's difficult, trying to find people at that right place. And spinal cord cases are delicate, and some people take a long time. You know, I've had cases that didn't get a job until that twelfth month. I have people who have never found a job. You know, to think it's going to be just a blanket fix, you know, it's not going to happen" (Smith-Morris et al. 2014: 148).

Identifying good job targets and then providing job leads or setting up interviews for participants was not enough to reach a positive employment outcome. The VR counselor had to discover participants' interests, maximize their readiness for job interviews and work, expand their capabilities through mechanical, technical, and clinical supports, and then discover possible sources for work to which the participant might apply. The process was invariably and intensively social, and its success depended on something that was hard to calibrate on a quantitative index: intensity of effort. This counselor was simultaneously a support counselor for the patient and an administrative assistant for setting up, and sometimes driving the veteran to, job interviews.

However, this absolutely radical approach to patient support shown by VR counselors in the SCI-VIP was sadly missed in the fidelity reporting that became the primary source of clinical information about what worked and did not work. Very little of this sort of ethnographic detail would find its way into the clinical publication of outcomes that were relied on to evaluate and promote this program with the government.

Competitive Employment

As a last example of the way qualitative evidence was pushed to the side in the evaluation exercises of the RCT and its publications, I turn to the case of competitive employment. Here the clinical publication offers a statement about the central metric of the trial's outcomes:

> Our primary outcome variable, employment, was defined as competitive employment obtained after the baseline interview. . . . Among the 201 subjects, 35 subjects (17.4%) accounted for 90 total jobs. The rate of employment for [Supported Employment] subjects was significantly greater (29.6%; 95% CI, 20.8–40.4) than that of either the TAU-IS[11] group (11.8%; 95% CI, 4.6–19.1; $P<.003$) or the TAU-OS[12] group (4.8%; 95% CI, 0.5–16.7; $P<.002$). When employment was restricted to competitive employment only, [Supported Employment] subjects significantly accounted for 50 (69.4%) of 72 jobs and were significantly more likely to achieve employment (25.9%; 95% CI, 17.6–36.5) compared with either TAU-IS subjects (10.5%; 95% CI, 3.6–17.4; $P<.008$) or TAU-OS subjects (2.3%; 95% CI, 0.0–12.9; $P<.002$). (Ottomanelli et al. 2012: 744)

The reduction of employment facts to a set of numerical figures about employment accomplishes a great deal for policymakers who want to show bottom lines in relation to employment statistics. Still we might ask if this sort of reporting also occludes the kinds of information that are of key importance to *understanding* how this program was able to achieve these indicators of program success in the first place.

Ethnographic materials that were gathered in the process of producing these numbers offer many more narrative terms and contextual detail, but they have great importance for the eventual replication of the trial's outcomes in clinical care, which is key to the VHA mission of blended research and clinical care. Ethnographic reports emphasize how the SCI-VIP adapted to each veteran's needs and readiness for employment. In fact despite their appearance of being similar when presented in numerical form, the specific services offered by the VR counselor were rarely consistent across veterans. Instead the VR counselor managed a caseload with a wide range of needs and readiness: securing interviews and job fitting for some, focusing on motivational interviewing with others. These varied widely from patient to patient, counselor to counselor. Take these kinds of statements from clients about what kinds of work would be meaningful or how they might obtain these jobs:

> We need purpose. And I know that I like feeling useful, not just to myself, I like to feel that I'm useful to society, to the country. That I can contribute in some small way, it's all of us working together to make the whole thing work. And of course, I feel useful. (Smith-Morris et al. 2013: 154)

> [This project] can't be made any better. It's just that they're reaching the people that they can reach. It's just up to them whether or not they want to better themselves by going back to work. (Smith-Morris unpublished research)

The veterans with spinal cord injuries became employed and the kinds of employment they found matched these sensibilities about what mattered in their relationships with VR counselors. Two examples of employed vets offer insight on this. One, Tim, was an online researcher and a payroll clerk. Another, Joe, found employment with a land title research company. Joe explained that his job consists of Internet research to inform land disputes and litigation. His work hours are flexible, and he works from home with minimal supervision and oversight. Joe states that he does some work in the morning or late at night, as he has ready access to the Internet. He considers the job ideal since the work does not interfere with his medical treatments and appointments. His notion of what mattered here (and why he could keep his job) were things that the VR counselor had to understand and take into consideration in her intervention efforts, and they reflected more fundamental concerns about how to be valuable to society.

Working in a similar environment, Tim is a payroll clerk for a company based in New Jersey (hundreds of miles away from his home). He explained that his work puts him in charge of verifying employee hours, calculating wages, and reporting to corporate offices—and he does all this from his home via the Internet. Much like Joe's, Tim's work schedule is fairly flexible, and he considers it the perfect fit for his life and needs. Again the VR counselor's ability to be attentive to diverse set of concerns, specific to each vet, was what made this employment trajectory successful. What is missed, then, in the streamlining and reducing of this information for CON-SORT and fidelity reporting, in the turning of these stories into numbers?

The ethnographic details about what kinds of jobs work, how to find them, and how to manage diverse caseloads that are attentive to individual client views of meaningful employment are integral to the program's success. Recognizing that these are precisely the kinds of details that are made invisible in reports that count, however, begs the question of not just fidelity (as in what kinds of things are evidence of successful program implementation) but reproducibility as well. Could other programs in other places really reproduce this success without knowing in detail *how* the VR counselor accomplished her goals? I turn now to consider what these evidentiary contrasts mean for the nation's most complex health care and research system.

Solemn Duty and the Politics of New Metrics

It would be far too simple to argue that quality monitoring and improvement are simple technologies of state domination or market exploitation. That is, quality monitoring and improvement are undoubtedly sites where the state enacts policies and where the market drives agendas (particularly cost-effectiveness). Given the depths to which quality and evidence-based rhetoric have penetrated and permeated the VHA system, we might consider how these practices work and what their broader effects are. As the VHA faces aggressive and cyclical political pressure to use taxpayer dollars wisely and to fulfill its "solemn duty" to care for those who "have borne the battle," we cannot underestimate the impact of the techniques for accounting and measuring what these programs accomplish.

The QUERI system is the VHA's "ambitious attempt to develop a data-driven national quality improvement program . . . to ensure excellence in all places where VHA provides health care services" (Demakis et al. 2000). The system is both a communicative system, conveying referential information, and an ideological system, deploying ideologies, political priorities, and administrative agendas through "collaborative links between researchers, clinicians, managers, and policy makers throughout different divisions with the organization" (118). Its modus operandi, however, is research. The eight steps of the QUERI process focus on the identification, definition, implementation, and documentation of "best practices," and it is in this "identification of best practices" (Step 2) that definitions of "quality" achieve hegemonic status. Through the trope of quality, biases and information choices are made invisible. Thus in Demakis et al., "quality" is aligned with a bodyless authority except to invoke the internationally powerful Institute of Medicine as corroborative in guideline decisions: "All [quality] guidelines and other evidence-based documents were assessed for quality (especially the rigor of the methods used during development and the degree to which the documentation explicitly states the strength of evidence underlying each recommendation) and also assessed for applicability to Veterans. The criteria developed by the Institute of Medicine were useful for this purpose" (122). Nowhere in this document is the concept of evidence explained or defined. Rather it is assumed to be found primarily in the numbers, through presumptions about scientific omniscience and objectivity via mechanisms like the CONSORT statement and the gold standard of the RCT.

In fact any reader familiar with clinical and health services literature of the past two decades knows well that the reference to quality implies little more than fidelity to the stage model for clinical outcome trials.[13] Here research modeled on the gold standard RCT offers the highest and best form of evidence for what works, what counts (Smith-Morris et al. 2014). For those of us doing ethnographic research, the question then remains: What happens to all that other evidence that falls outside the RCT model? For the VHA's QUERI system, this problem is summed up in a dismissive phrase: "Although process and structural data are also needed, outcome measurement is prioritized" (Demakis et al. 2000: 123). Indeed the transition of the VHA toward evidence-based clinical care and clinical trial research is described as a "maturation of the health services research field" (123). But what kind of maturation is this, and what kinds of obfuscations are entailed in making these measurements possible?

I am eager to point out that the VHA and its QUERI system have at times relied on ethnographic data (what Demakis et al. 2000 called "structural and process data") to do the work of measuring the impact of trials and outcome research. Volume 37 of the *Annals of Anthropological Practice* was dedicated to ethnographic work within the VA system, and is a robust testimony to the relevance of ethnographic data for clinical trials. But it is also clear that these "structural and process data" find limited room in policy and clinical publications. They are not part of CONSORT requirements. Journals carrying these data are less valorized (lower impact factors, lower science indices), and the social scientists producing them are not typically invited to working groups that design both research and treatment guidelines (Adams 2002, 2005; Smith-Morris 2015). Hammell (2007: 271) confirmed this in finding that "surprisingly little research has explicitly sought to explore the experience of rehabilitation following SCI."

The limited room for qualitative data is important and notable, but it is not the only problem. Simple inclusion of qualitative data in or alongside quantitative reports is insufficient since the decision-making power, resource allocation, and professional hierarchies of clinical work profoundly impact care *and* the way that research is conducted. The truths about program effectiveness are found in critical examination not only of the trial and its interventions and outcomes but also in the dynamic relationships among humans and within institutions through which RCTs are enacted (Nguyen 2010; Petryna 2009). Thus although anthropological tools and methods can be attached to outcomes research, it is clear that quantitative research has a better chance of being recognized and influential in the places that matter.

The VHA example parallels the large-scale, state investments in middle- and low-income country health care and allows us to extend this conversation of "which metrics matter" into global health. Nguyen's (2010: 91) "therapeutic citizenship" encompasses the activism, knowledge about potentially better treatments, and "a sense of political engagement" that gay activists in South Africa developed over access to HIV medications. Demanding first access to participate in RCTs, and later to the medications themselves, this generation of activist patients conceptualized their targets as *rights* and the duty of the state to ensure them. The VHA as a government body is vulnerable to the same politicized pressures — although this pressure does not always emerge from patient groups. Instead the VHA responds to superior political and governmental offices, to external stakeholders and competitors for federal funds ($589 million requested for 2015), to their own veteran members, and ultimately to the voting citizenry.

Nguyen's (2010) therapeutic citizens and Petryna's (2009) biological citizens emerged as influential only after they became organized, informed, and politicized. In both of these cases organization cohered around a particular diagnosis or related syndrome of problems. Even in these diagnostically related groups, however, membership in the groups is heterogeneous. On their way to heterodoxic status, groups advocating health *rights* claim converts from the margins of orthodox medicine. Similarly Davis and Nichter (2015) address how biomedical doctors who are friendly to the calls for holistic and chronic attention to Lyme disease add legitimacy and force to therapeutic citizenship. Indeed social scientists who work alongside RCTs (as in my work) or in "health partnerships" to support clinicians (e.g., in Haiti; see Minn, this volume) may offer one way of interjecting contextualized data and metrics into global health.

But, as Taussig (1980) and others have warned, these collaborations are fraught. Political aims in a variety of global contexts are regularly legitimized through quantitative metrics. I return to Demakis et al.'s (2000: 123) comment about the VHA, that the "maturation" of a health science research "field" is tied to "evidence-based clinical care and clinical trial research." This strategic phraseology envisions a "field" that is first about methods of quantification and objectification, not about clear and full understanding of the results of interventions. A "field" built on metrics that include only quantities and ignore scientific evidence that resists quantification is a house of cards: a thin-walled, unstable, and hollow structure. While the benefits of RCT methodology and evidence gathering are not disputed, the gap between outcomes and the contextual evidence that explains those outcomes is wide and growing (Adams 2002, 2005; Adams et al. 2005; Smith-Morris et al. 2014). My fear is that qualitative research seems to have lost the battle for health care and federal-funding relevance.

The legitimization of political aims through scientific metrics allows a variety of actors to claim both moral and scientific authority. Better global health will require both better metrics and ethnographic engagement, social scientific evidence, and a tolerance for the small scale—not always seeking economies of scale. In their comprehensive discussion of poverty alleviation, Banerjee and Duflo (2011) argue that to influence health care, one must understand health-seeking behavior; that top-down health policies (e.g., mandated prevention behaviors) are a costly waste of time in some environments; and that there are "deep reasons" (154) and "time inconsistencies" (194) that de-link truly effective health care from any single strategy, no matter how well evidenced and supported by RCT metrics.[14]

The greater dilemma for global health that an obsession with metrics will create is what David Armstrong (1995) calls "surveillance medicine." Just as colonial medicine controlled the brown and black hordes through pathologization of their bodies and identities, surveillance medicine problematizes normality, redrawing the relationships among symptom, sign, and illness and using medicine's newest tools—its evidentiary forms, including the RCT and CONSORT guidelines—to define risk and moralize conformity. Biehl and Petryna's (2013) more recent volume does an excellent job of exposing this new species of health surveillance in the name of better governance.

With all this winning, maturation, and quality at our fingertips, it is a wonder that VHA secretaries still rotate in and out with regular swings of the political pendulum. Arguably this is because the environment is shifting as well as the citizenry. The VHA as an institution claims to serve the *rights* of veterans to receive health care and to enjoy the benefits of well-funded, scientific investigatory efforts. The VHA therefore harnesses some of the same tropes of therapeutic citizenship as the people it serves! It is beyond this discussion to dissect the hierarchy of power and political influence that yields any given VHA budget. Suffice it to say that the QUERI program represents one successful director's agenda: with the ideologies, symbols, goals, targets, methods, promises, and strategies that were not only institutionally achievable but were also popular in the media-informed public. The evidence-based agenda will continue to propel a diversity of agendas because it is the trope that works.

Ethnographic and qualitative data must catalyze their own therapeutic citizenship. In defense and promotion of qualitative data, a number of authors (Biehl and Petryna 2013; Sobo 2009) remind us of the power of the idiosyncratic story to capture a reading public's imagination. We might also ask how this sort of work bolsters our sensibilities to what counts, to what is reliable, valid, and analytically powerful. Qualitative researchers will continue to narrate local and idiosyncratic lessons from the field, but we must also claim relevance in the highly structured world of intervention trials and evidence-based care. It is the job of social critics to be mindful of the myriad and sometimes unquantifiable forces acting in "evidence" production, especially in places that are under the rationed funding and bureaucratic supervision of governments.

Notes

1. There are even studies on the quality of the Total Quality Management approach and of programs that purport to employ the approach, in a disorienting circular system of reference (e.g., Lammers et al. 1996).

2. Indeed the transformation was actually based on a "value equation, in which value is considered to be a function of technical quality, access to care, patient functional status, and services satisfaction all divided by the cost or price of the care" (Kizer and Dudley 2008: 18.5).

3. It should not be surprising that the man who by many accounts accomplished the needed transformation was described as "a dynamic policy entrepreneur" (Oliver 2007: 15).

4. U.S. Department of Veterans Affairs, "Funding," accessed November 2, 2014, http://www.research.va.gov/funding.

5. The VHA Office of Research and Development is divided into four parts: Biomedical Laboratory R&D, Clinical Services R&D, Health Services R&D, and Rehabilitation R&D. The $589 million budget request is labeled "medical and prosthetic research," while another $59 billion is requested for "medical care" for eligible veterans.

6. See Gary Marcus and Ernest Davis, op-ed "Eight (No Nine!) Problems With Big Data," *New York Times*, April 6, 2014.

7. My role as a limited-time contractor speaks to the marginalized market position of many qualitative researchers within the VHA system. McCullough et al. (2013) have written about the tenuousness of this type of contract for professionals (especially those without university affiliations) whose scholarly expertise is drained by a contract employment system because it does not allow time for, or even necessarily see the value of, publication and engagement within the larger anthropological community. The contract labor format facilitates an agile, relatively inexpensive, and constantly fresh supply of expert researchers in any given location. But the format is unstable, professionally draining, and intellectually parasitic for scholars whose continuing expertise depends in part on an ongoing nurturing of methodological, theoretical, professional, and topical learning exclusive to their degree-granting field, something categorically difficult to obtain in contract work (McCullough et al. 2013; Bowman et al. 2008).

8. Including the weekly meetings of all vocational rehabilitation (VR) counselors, the VIP VR counselor conference calls, the VIP site coordinator conference calls, and the Inter-Disciplinary Team meetings.

9. Fidelity to the Supported Employment model was measured in a number of ways. The program records of SCI-VIP as well as participant medical records are reviewed biannually to assess the degree to which the program (documented in these notes) adheres to the principles of evidence-based Supported Employment described by Bond 2004. During site visits consultant trainers gather data on program fidelity through semistructured interviews with consumers, employers, clinicians, program managers, health care team members, administrative management and leadership; chart reviews; and observation of team meetings. A fidelity scale for Supported Employment, which has been widely used and is consistently linked with employment outcomes among

programs that serve persons with mental illness, was also used in SCI-VIP (Becker et al. 2001; Bond et al. 2008a).

10. There were eight principles. Please see Bond et al. (2001) for details.

11. Therapy As Usual—Interventional Site.

12. Therapy As Usual—Observational Site.

13. U.S. Food and Drug Administration, "The FDA's Drug Review Process: Ensuring Drugs Are Safe and Effective," November 6, 2014, http://www.fda.gov/drugs/resourcesforyou/consumers/ucm143534.htm.

14. That is, the psychological difficulty of matching our actions today with our vision for the future.

9 · THE TYRANNY OF THE WIDGET An American Medical Aid Organization's Struggles with Quantification PIERRE MINN

In 1939 the General Motors Corporation created a six-minute animated film to explain economic processes to children. Entitled *Round and Round* the film focuses on a factory that produces "widgets." The widgets appear as nondescript cubes, and the narrator tells us, "A widget might be a radio, a refrigerator, a musical instrument, or a motor car. A widget, you know, is just symbol for any manufactured product that people use." As the story unfolds, the widget maker sells his widgets to a farmer, a coal miner, a steel manufacturer, and a lumberman. These individuals in turn sell their raw materials to the widget maker. Money circulates in one direction, widgets in the other. The result, according to the film, is a harmonious circle of exchanges. By using "widgets," the filmmakers direct their young viewers' attention away from the specificities, intentions, or results of exchanges. The focus is on the process of exchanges rather than their particularities or contents.[1]

Seven decades later the director of a small American medical aid NGO used the term *widget* in a more disparaging manner. Nathan Nickerson directs Konbit Sante, an organization based in Portland, Maine, that operates health programs in northern Haiti. Konbit Sante works in partnership with Haiti's public health sector, supporting the work of Haitian health care workers rather than directly implementing clinical interventions. Describing their challenges in obtaining funding, Nickerson told me, "Funders want to know how many widgets you've given out — we just don't work that way." While the widgets in the General Motors film appeared as valuable objects, useful to and desired by all, for Nickerson they represented a unit that was often alien to his organization's mission but that had to be taken seriously because of its valence among those who could provide resources and support.

While the dynamics I describe here relate specifically to an American organization's activities in Haiti, many are relevant to other aid projects that operate across other contexts of marked inequalities and disparities. In the broader realms of international development and intervention, new programs and policies stress integrated projects, sustainability, and capacity building, and many organizations and aid bodies face the challenges of reconciling their missions and operations with the exigencies of funders and donors (Bornstein 2005; Escobar 2011; Ferguson 1994). The emergence of the term *donor-driven*, generally to designate an undesirable attribute, has emerged in the past three decades to draw attention to the misalignment between donors' priorities and approaches and the needs and operations of recipients and intermediaries. These divides are particularly evident in the realm of transnational health projects, which link markedly different social and economic realms: for example, a one-room clinic in northern Haiti and USAID offices in Washington, DC. They are also accentuated by the wide range of programs, target objects, and instruments that constitute health interventions, ranging from clinical encounters to disease prevention and infrastructure development. Given the discrepancies between the working conditions and operations that can exist between these two categories of actors, it is not surprising that divides occur in relation to fundamental issues of temporality and classification.

This chapter describes the strategies Konbit Sante staff and volunteers, particularly the group's U.S. leadership, use to communicate their interventions to current and prospective funders. Many of the group's core principles and primary activities lie outside the purview of (and at times come into direct conflict with) the values and priorities of the group's supporters, which include private and governmental funding bodies, individual donors, and media that describes the organization and its activities. These discrepancies are indicative of misalignments in two general areas. The first is the temporality of aid and expectations for when the final outcomes of the interventions should occur. The second involves ownership of data and what impact this ownership has on the quality of numbers produced and the purposes they serve.

In considering these misalignments, it is important to stress that Konbit Sante's leadership demonstrates no resistance or reticence to the idea that the group should be accountable for its engagements, either to the populations it serves or to its supporters and funders. In addition to preparing the requisite detailed reports and analyses that are integral to contemporary funding structures, the organization maintains an active and detailed website that chronicles its activities and progress. In my own work studying Konbit Sante, I have found its staff and volunteers to be exceptionally open to and interested in perspectives and processes that could improve the organization's functioning and impact. The problem therefore lies not in funders' demands for accountability and transparency but in the limited scope and rigid nature of the units and terms that are being used to evaluate global health interventions. In a similar vein Konbit Sante's members do not minimize the importance or necessity of working with quantitative health indicators such as vaccine rates or maternal mortality. Rather they (like many informants whose voices are heard throughout this volume) stress that these indicators are insufficient for evaluating the overall strength of a health system and, when taken out of context or used exclusively, can present a skewed portrait of health conditions and services.

I first encountered Konbit Sante while conducting ethnographic research on international medical aid in northern Haiti from 2007 to 2009. Most of my study focused on the Hôpital Universitaire Justinien (HUJ), a 250-bed public hospital in Haiti's second largest city, Cap-Haïtien. Although there are several dozen international organizations and governmental agencies that implement a variety of programs in the hospital (e.g., donating shipments of medical supplies, sending teams of clinicians to carry out specialized surgeries, subsidizing care for pregnant women and infants), Konbit Sante was one of the most prominent groups. The organization was frequently referred to by the hospital's administration as "our privileged partners" and almost always named first when I asked the hospital staff to name the foreign groups and organizations that were present in their hospital. I also interviewed Konbit Sante staff and volunteers and carried out observations and participant observations at the group's meeting with hospital leadership and employees, at trainings they conducted for hospital staff, and informally at meals, discussions, and other activities in the Cap-Haïtien area. I visited the organization's headquarters in Maine on two occasions, before beginning my research in 2006 and in the summer of 2008.

A growing body of anthropological research focuses on the work and roles of so-called local health care workers in impoverished settings (Closser 2010; Wendland 2010). While much of my research focused on the interactions between foreign aid projects and Haitian clinical staff, here I focus primarily on data gathered from Konbit Sante's U.S. staff and leadership. This focus brings into relief the processes through which actors at a particular node in a larger sequence of aid solicitations, negotiations, and transfers struggle to make their work "count" in the calculus of individuals and organizations deciding where to distribute financial resources.

Medical Missions

Konbit Sante's foundation and genesis are indicative of tendencies in the sphere of transnational medical and humanitarian aid in the millennial period. These include the ongoing proliferation of NGOs, struggles and deliberation over the role of the state in the provision of health services, and a focus on a new series of priorities in health and development interventions: health systems strengthening, sustainability, and capacity building (Minn 2011; Schuller 2012; Wubneh 2003). While these priorities and strategies are officially espoused by the organizations that shape international health policies and distribute aid resources, they are also sources of friction and tension as small organizations such as Konbit Sante seek to obtain grants and donations in what appears to be an increasingly competitive aid market.

Konbit Sante's official institutional biography states that it was created in 2000 by a group of Portland health professionals who were seeking to contribute to improving the health of an impoverished population. In interviews with the group's early members and volunteers, I learned that many of them had been engaged in transnational medical aid projects. Some had participated in week-long medical missions, in which North

American clinical teams — often affiliated with Christian churches — travel to rural and impoverished areas and provide consultations and treatments in makeshift clinics (usually in schools or churches). Many of these teams maintain relationships with local religious leaders or prominent community members and return annually with stocks of basic medications and other supplies. Medical missions are particularly widespread in Haiti and other parts of the Caribbean and Latin America, due to the region's proximity to the United States and Canada, which allows for short-term travel and interventions.

Several of Konbit Sante's members who had participated repeatedly in such medical missions in Latin America and Africa eventually grew frustrated with that model of care. They felt that the needs in the communities they visited were enormous and reflected a lack of access to even basic primary care, and it became frustrating for them to see the same conditions (and in some cases the same individuals) year after year with no visible improvement in the population's health conditions. Dr. Michael Taylor, a charismatic dermatologist with a background in public health, founded the group in 2000. His approach is described as follows on the organization's website: "[Dr. Taylor] questioned the value of having foreign doctors come into a community for a short time, provide care, then leave without ensuring a health system is in place for patients in need tomorrow, the next day, and into the future. 'There must be a better way to use the resources and talent of the Greater Portland community to make a difference,' he remembers thinking. Dr. Taylor and his wife, Wendy Taylor, found others with similar experiences and beliefs and they began planning."[2]

Before describing the alternative model Konbit Sante's founders developed, it is important to note several dimensions of short-term medical missions that are relevant to issues of metrics and quantification. I accompanied and observed several of these week-long medical missions during my fieldwork in Haiti and found that quantification was central to their activities. For the groups that traveled to rural areas to offer primary care consultations, their goal was to bring the largest team possible to Haiti while remaining able to manage logistics for the groups (housing, transportation, translators' services, etc.). In a school-based clinic, groups were divided into smaller teams based on professional specialization and assigned a local translator to assist in communicating with patients. After their first missions, groups had generally devised a rudimentary system of patient files (or at least registration forms), which allowed them to keep track of the number of patients seen, medications distributed, equipment dispensed, and referrals made. These numbers, particularly those of patients seen, were often inscribed on a chalkboard near the group's dining area so that members could keep track of them over the course of the week. After the missions were completed, numbers would again play an important role in reporting activities to supporting communities. Here are three typical examples taken from medical mission trip reports and newsletters:

> Our team consisted of 26 members working in the specialties of dentistry, gynecology, pediatrics, and adult medicine. We had a fully functioning pharmacy in 2 locations staffed by a licensed pharmacist. We spent 4 days in Chantal and divided the team in half so 2 days could be spent in Canon Haiti. Each day we saw approximately 400–600 patients. We were supported by 22 staff members including 5 laboratory technicians, interpreters, security guards, cooks and drivers." —Juliet Geiger, RN, We Care to Share[3]

2012 TRIP STATISTICS:
- Deworming program implemented in the small remote village (Jeanty) in the city of Grand-goave [sic], Haiti.
- 1331 school-aged children were dewormed.
- 2-seater latrine built (projected to last 20 years).
- 500 pairs of shoes, sneakers, and sandals delivered to school-aged children as part of deworming program.
- Over 2,000 toothbrushes delivered in concert with hygiene education on sanitation.
- More than $47,000 worth of medical supplies and equipment delivered.

—Rowlens Melduni, MD, Clinicians of the World[4]

We provided medical care to 516 patients: 344 in primary care in mobile clinics + 64 dental patients treated for tooth decay and abscess, 3 patients at the general hospital in Port-au-Prince (PaP) evaluated for mastectomy and continuing oncologic care and 105 patients treated at HSC [Hôpital Ste-Croix]. 21 surgeries were done at HSC — 9 major and 12 minor. We treated 329 adults and 187 children. Ground work [sic] was laid at FSIL [a nursing school] for a long term women's health study with faculty. Preoperative teaching was videotaped for the mastectomy patients to use in future cases. —Lisa Kerr Johnson,

PharmD, Haiti Medical Mission, First Presbyterian Church of Ann Arbor[5]

The categories listed (patients seen, medications dispensed, procedures carried out) represent the most common metrics for short-term medical mission groups. This type of calculus fits well with the practice of biomedicine, where patients' bodies and clinicians' therapies are seen as discrete, enumerable entities. It is also visible in the context of other types of material aid interventions: books delivered, plows distributed, houses built, and trees planted. While these types of interventions bring material and health resources into remote areas where they are sorely needed, they have also been criticized for the disruption they cause in the communities where they occur, as well as for the ways they undermine other institutions that are perennially active in these communities (Hefferan 2007; Wainwright 2001). As Nickerson told me, "The numbers of pounds or volume of supplies or medicines are often cited, for example, without specifying what is actually needed or desired. Unless these numbers are more fully contextualized, they can be very misleading."

Understanding the work of short-term, clinical medical missions and the quantifications they use to describe and represent their interventions is crucial for understanding Konbit Sante, its model and its activities. Despite the fact that the organization's founders were explicit in their critique of conventional medical mission approaches, its leaders and members must consistently differentiate Konbit Sante's work to potential supporters, who assume that the group is premised on facilitating Americans' clinical interventions in Haiti. The main reason for this is the prominence and visibility of clinical missions: while the exact number of organizations carrying out these interventions in Haiti is unknown, they are active throughout the country and receive particular prominence in local media and through faith-based networks and professional organizations. Members of medical missions often practice fundraising at the community level, which increases the visibility of their actions in ways that grant-based funding does not. In addition the prominence of larger organizations such as Médecins sans frontières and the International Committee of the Red Cross (while very different in scope and content from smaller medical missions) also promote the image of mobile, northern clinicians tending to patients in the South, this despite the much higher numbers of "local" staff involved in these organizations (Redfield 2013). Finally, it is arguable whether the quantifiable nature of these interventions—patients seen, medicine distributed, surgeries performed—contributes to the visibility and prominence of this style of intervention. These discrete procedures and the numbers that quantify them are easily communicated and easily understood without knowledge of the contexts in which they occur.

The members of Konbit Sante, however, must not only explain to supporters and potential supporters that their work does not correspond to expectations about medical intervention in a country like Haiti; they must also describe a partnership that is difficult to quantify, that is legible only in light of the geographic, social, and economic context in which it is situated, and that can change rather quickly in its outward manifestations and operations, even if the underlying values and principles that guide them remain consistent.

Building a Health Partnership

Recently Nickerson asked me if I would be able to suggest an "elevator speech" for Konbit Sante board members to describe the organization. He explained that the members often struggled to describe the organization to outsiders and that my years of following Konbit Sante as an anthropologist might give me a unique perspective on their work. Anthropologists are better known for expanding and lengthening messages than reducing them, but in the end I offered a message with three components that seemed to capture the organization's essence and distinctiveness:[6]

1   Konbit Sante is a small health NGO that focuses its activities in northern Haiti, in and around the city of Cap-Haïtien (Haiti's second largest city).
2   The organization partners directly with Haiti's public health sector, specifically the Ministry of Public Health and Population.
3   Instead of directly implementing clinical interventions, the organization focuses on supporting Haitian staff.

The issues of quantification and metrics is particularly relevant to the third component, but can also be considered in light of the first two.

Operating in a peripheral urban area comes with a particular set of challenges. Many medical aid groups in Haiti intervene in rural areas, dispensing services in villages and hamlets with populations in the hundreds or low thousands. While Haiti's high population density and the mobility of rural

Haitians (particularly to access medical care and other scarce resources) make the specific numbers associated with administrative areas less significant in reality, groups working in rural areas will nonetheless be able to produce impressive statistics that aspire to convey efficacy and achievement (e.g., "We consulted over four hundred patients in a village of twelve hundred people"). Working in the city of Cap-Haïtien, whose population is estimated to be as high as 700,000, Konbit Sante will see its quantifiable interventions diluted due to the number of people in its targeted polity. On the other hand, Konbit Sante does not operate on a national level, as do most international organizations and agencies, who are able to draw upon the Haiti-wide scope of their efforts to claim the impact of their programs on all of Haiti's citizenry, whether in the form of prevention messages, national policies, or other countrywide campaigns.

Its partnership with Haiti's government has also impacted the ways Konbit Sante relates to numbers and quantitative metrics. One the one hand, data collection is a prominent feature in Haiti's public clinical sites. Its most visible manifestation is in the form of clinic and hospital staff, generally nurses, who are charged with collecting patients' demographic information and vital statistics prior to consultations and procedures. This information is laboriously copied into thick ledgers that, in the case of most facilities, are stacked on a bookshelf or cabinet to accumulate dust. While a privately owned or operated facility would have greater control over the collection and use of data, the hospital and clinic where Konbit Sante operates its programs do not have strong or centralized systems for ensuring the quality of the information collected, compiling or analyzing statistics, or applying the data to solve health-related problems. While information technologies and data infrastructures seem to be improving the situation (particularly in relation to infectious disease reporting and maternal and child health), partnering with government institutions means that Konbit Sante is unable to provide the types of reliable metrics and data that other NGOs are more easily able to obtain, process, and communicate.

These obstacles would be frustrating enough if Konbit Sante's goal were to produce evidence of quantifiable interventions. On a deeper level, however, the organization's leadership struggles with the fact that its very goal of strengthening Haiti's public health care system is particularly difficult, if not impossible, to quantify. Nickerson frequently gives two examples to illustrate this point. The first relates to a moment after the devastating 2010 earthquake, when the HUJ was inundated with offers of assistance from dozens of foreign groups and organizations. While Cap-Haïtien is located far from the quake's epicenter and there was no structural damage or casualties in the region, the hospital's directors were overwhelmed with the enormity of the catastrophe, which involved personal and family losses, an influx of patients fleeing the earthquake zone, and an interruption of nearly all basic routines and transactions. It was at this time that the hospital's medical director asked Konbit Sante to coordinate all of the offers of foreign assistance for the institution. In a context where international aid represents a crucial component in hospital's basic functioning and where caution and discretion in managing incoming and potential resources is paramount, the trust and rapport involved in delegating this responsibility to a foreign organization cannot be overstated. Konbit Sante took on this responsibility for several months before convincing the hospital's administrators that they themselves were able to reassume their coordinating role.

The second example involves the hospital's new executive director, who took on this role in 2012. This physician, the hospital's only urologist, inherited an extremely stressful position that involved resource allocation and decisions regarding personnel and hospital policies. This physician had maintained close working ties with Konbit Sante since the group's creation, working with Maine physicians to develop the hospital's urology department, traveling to Portland for stints at Maine Medical Center, and seeking support in the forms of material donations and training. Shortly after he assumed the role of executive director, he approached Konbit Sante's leaders and asked them to undertake a full and frank assessment of the hospital's financial management practices, with the goal of increasing the institution's accountability and transparency. This would involve revealing particularly sensitive information about the hospital, its operations, and its staff.

In both of these cases Konbit Sante's U.S. members took these gestures as signs of the trust and positive rapport that existed between them and the hospital's management, and of the transparency and courage of certain members of the hospital's administration. I heard Nickerson mention on several occasions that he had never heard of a government health establishment that offered this level of unfettered access to a foreign organization. Based on my own experiences of studying medical aid in Haiti, I can concur that this level of divulging information is remarkable. Haitian health professionals and administrators, despite their privileged place in Haitian society, occupy relatively subordinate positions in the world of international medical aid. They are often considered implementers rather than allocators and decision makers, and those who occupy leadership roles (such as hospital directors) are extremely cautious and discrete when it comes to interactions with foreign aid bodies, playing their cards very close to their chests.

These two examples allowed Konbit Sante to intervene in very concrete ways (such as coordinating earthquake relief efforts and helping improve budgeting practices), but more important for the organization's leadership, they were positive signs of all the work that had been done in previous years to build confidence and an egalitarian partnership. "But how," Nickerson asked me rhetorically, "can you quantify this? There's no line in the funders' reports where you can give them a measure of the trust that's been built over the years."

In many ways simply working with government structures, which in Haiti are associated with complex bureaucracy, long delays, and a generalized opacity of procedures, could be considered a form of achievement. While international observers lament nongovernmental and other parallel systems that have weakened state structures worldwide, and some governments (notably, that of Rwanda) have been more successful in requiring aid organizations to cooperate with state structures, organizations like Konbit Sante often find that calls for increased collaboration with public health systems are not always rewarded by systems that allocate resources and funding. The presence of such tensions in widely disparate settings (see Smith-Morris, Hales, both this volume) indicates that struggles to reconcile emerging health metrics and the specificities of particular interventions and programs are as widespread and global as global health itself.

While these domains illustrate some of Konbit Sante's challenges in communicating its activities in quantifiable terms, tensions are most visible in light of the group's commitment to supporting Haitian clinicians and institutions rather than implementing their own clinical interventions. This area also brings into relief issues of systemic approaches and temporality, highlighting fundamental differences in conceptions and programs of resolutions for an ailing and impoverished population.

Supporting Haitian Clinicians

When Konbit Sante's founders decided in the early 2000s that they would not focus on the provision of clinical services, they were part of a larger trend in transnational medical projects that emphasized the importance of so-called local health care workers in the provision of health services to impoverished populations. The 2006 World Health Report, entitled *Working Together for Health*, focused on the "global health workforce," addressing issues such as shortages of health professionals, emigration, and training (World Health Organization 2006). The report is filled with predictions of the negative consequences resulting from too few nurses, physicians, midwives, and other health professionals, particularly in the Global South. In Haiti's case many of these predictions are already a reality, with serious shortages at all levels of clinicians, a concentration of health professionals and specialists in the Port-au-Prince area (leaving most of the country without access), and high rates of international emigration (Dubois et al. 2007).

At its most basic level Konbit Sante's support of Haitian staff involves sponsoring salaries for Haitian clinicians and health agents embedded in the public health care system. An early example of this was the hiring of attending physicians in internal medicine and pediatrics, whose responsibilities would include training and supervising medical residents in these services. At the time the HUJ was one of only two sites in the country where medical graduates could complete a three- or four-year residency. Supervision and real mentorship, however, were sorely lacking. Nearly all attending physicians in Haitian public hospitals operate private clinics. While some balance their hours between their public appointments and private employment, the majority are seldom present in the public institutions. During my fourteen months at the hospital I met only a small minority of attending physicians officially appointed at the establishment. For what are often ambiguously referred to as "political reasons," it is virtually impossible to fire a government physician; doctors receive their (admittedly small: US$500 per month) checks regardless of their presence on the job.

In this context residents seeking training and supervision are left with relatively few options. As they are prohibited from performing any work outside their institution of residency, many simply turn to each other for guidance and mentorship. At the time Konbit Sante began its partnership in Cap-Haïtien, the Pediatrics Department at the hospital (one of the largest in the country) had a single resident. The organization decided to sponsor the salary of two attending physicians, both of whom maintained private clinics and worked with other NGOs, but required that they register a specific number of hours at HUJ and implement a complete training course for the residents, including a morning report, rounds, and individual supervision. By the time I finished my fieldwork in 2009 the number of residents had increased to sixteen, and today they number over twenty-five. Konbit Sante's pediatric staff also includes a nurse educator who works to improve the quality of education in the hospital's affiliated nursing school and acts as a liaison and mentor for student nurses on rotation in the pediatric service.

When this intervention is reported to donors and funders, the hiring of two physicians and a nurse educator can appear quite minimal in numeric terms. Even the number of residents, whose expansion as a percentage is quite remarkable, remains quite low in sheer numbers. However, Konbit Sante considers its partnership with the Pediatrics Department to be one of its most successful initiatives. While the training has been accompanied by major infrastructure projects in and material donations to the pediatrics services, the training of residents remains a flagship intervention in that service, and perhaps in the hospital more broadly. Perhaps because its leaders know that the results of the program may not be particularly impressive when expressed in quantitative terms, the program is most often described with emphases on the passion, dedication, and talent of the sponsored attending physicians.

In supporting training initiatives, Konbit Sante's staff work with the aspiration that trainees will remain in Haiti to offer clinical services and increase provider-patient ratios in the country. They are keys actors in a health system that has yet to be built, one that the organization's leaders speak of in terms of a distant future. Both formal and informal projections run counter to positive projections. Current rates of international emigration by Haitian professionals are estimated to be 85 percent, and health professionals are no exception (Mattoo et al. 2005). Of the fifty-two medical residents at HUJ that I interviewed in 2009, only two stated that they intended to remain in Haiti upon completing their residency. Even before emigration the move to private health care establishments has drained the public system of personnel (Batha 2011).

The issue of international emigration is not mentioned in Konbit Sante's online materials and annual reports, although they are acutely aware of this transnational process and of the impediments it creates for ensuring decent quality of care. Some of the organization's Haitian staff and trainees have left Haiti to pursue careers abroad. The issue also becomes a topic of discussion and debate when the organization's members invite Haitian staff and colleagues for visits or internships in Maine. I heard several of the group's American members wonder if these visits and the exposure they gave to working environments and living conditions in a relatively affluent U.S. community fueled their Haitian guests' desires to emigrate and ended up working against the organization's goals. Conversely several of Konbit Sante's former employees now occupy positions of influence in both the public and private sectors in Haiti. Nickerson noted that "investing in helping professionals be successful in the country is another intangible benefit" of Konbit Sante's model.

Responding to Pressures to Quantify

The dynamics I have described are not concealed or implicit for the members of Konbit Sante. Particularly in the case of the organization's leadership and most active members (including board members, who have been acting as intermediaries between Haitian clinical sites and international funders for years), they are able to clearly articulate the tensions between funders' exigencies related to reporting and metrics and the organization's values and goals. Nickerson described these tensions in this fashion:

> Most funding is about counting the outputs, minimally, whether you're talking about the numbers of people getting vaccinated or the numbers of pre-natal visits or whatever. . . . And that's what, by and large, people pay for, and are looking for: evidence of the cost-effectiveness, or cost-benefit, or any one of those terms, that their dollar is actually producing, in a relatively rapid fashion, a turnaround on the investment, that's a deliverable on the ground. So I think that's some of the tension that we've felt, that, yes, you can do that, run a program and vaccinate a lot of people, but if your goal is really to work over time with the people that are here so that their system is better able to deliver that with less outside help, the first deliverables aren't that, necessarily. So I think that's where some of the tension has been. We've often felt like a square peg in a round hole.

Nickerson, who holds a doctorate in public health and is also a registered nurse, is quick to explain that he is not opposed to quantitative measures:

> I am sympathetic to the idea, as some people have said, "Well, what are the measures of building capacity, then unless it shows that those things are being delivered better, that that is the final measure of capacity building. If you're saying that you're helping them do it better,

then it ought to be the same outcome, then you should be seeing it on the ground." A lot of it is more tied into the time frame. It's not a linear where you pay for this to get done . . . it's more building something, it's more complicated with real capacity building. It's hard to find those indices, and in fact some of the more qualitative work is probably more appropriate to that kind of measure. So from my point of view, we really do want to know outcomes, if it's actually doing any good and if mortality rates are dropping as a result of work in these partnerships and efforts. It's just a couple of steps further down the logic frame.

Temporality is at the heart of this conflict. While the funding cycles of most donors involve annual or, at most, five-year calendars and deadlines, Konbit Sante's model of strengthening a health care system has a more expansive time frame, where progress and achievements in quantifiable form may not be apparent in time for the next reporting deadline or grant cycle.

While Konbit Sante's activities do not easily lend themselves to measurement using quantitative tools, this does not mean that the organization does not participate in quantitative data collection. In fact collecting these data is a time-consuming activity for the group's Haitian staff, particularly its program managers. Konbit Sante's U.S.-based program specialist, Tezita Negussie, describes the work of Haitian staff who oversee a community health outreach program in a peripheral clinic:

[The Haitian program managers] have really focused on, to the exclusion of everything else, on the USAID projects and spend enormous amounts of time and energy making sure that we are meeting those numbers objectives set by USAID, and have spent very little time on any of the other projects. So although we may have set objectives for the projects we were able to do through smaller grants, they haven't been taken as seriously and haven't had the same kind of attention that USAID receives. . . . USAID expects monthly reports, they expect trimestral reports, they do site visits, we are constantly monitored by them, and that's where our biggest source of funding comes from. So the expectations are higher and the money is more, so that's where the attention immediately goes to.

Even more than Nickerson, Negussie is quick to emphasize that collecting quantitative metrics is not a problem. In fact she wishes that Konbit Sante as an organization was more committed to measuring its activities and outcomes, whether through quantitative or qualitative measures. She doesn't believe that USAID is being unreasonable in its demands for data; rather the problem lies in the administrative structures that shape its collection and compilation:

> In all cases except for ours, the facilities that are funded by this project are run by the NGO. . . . That's not the case with us. So our program managers, in order to fill out all the paperwork, have to go to [the peripheral clinic] and get these numbers from different staff, and these staff members feel put upon, feel like their time is wasted, and don't understand why they're doing something for which they are not being paid, that takes up tons of time.

As mentioned earlier, data collection in Haitian clinical sites is considered a tedious and onerous task. In public sites data may be painstakingly collected for reports to the establishment's administration or the Ministry of Health, but the ledgers themselves generally do not leave the site. As even major clinical sites often lack functioning photocopiers, data for the reports described earlier must be laboriously copied by hand.

Even if Negussie and Nickerson do not always agree on the place that metrics and quantification should have in the organization, both emphasize that the question of data ownership is fundamental. Data in Haitian hospitals and clinics can serve different purposes; however, it most often seems to be generated with an outside authority in mind rather than for internal use. Most large funding agencies require detailed (but primarily numerical) data related to the activities they support. When I visit Haitian clinical sites, it is not uncommon for staff to hand me the ledger to examine. The information these ledgers reveal, however, is generally enumerative rather than synthesizing, and I suspect that the display is intended to convey a commitment to the process of data collection rather than information about the patients or services at the site.

While data collection, often associated with government agencies and religious communities, has a long history in Haiti (Bordes 1992, 1997), the use of data by those charged with collecting it is not widespread. More often than not, the data are collected for someone else, whether a government office in Port-au-Prince, an international funder, or as part of a visiting researcher's team. A comprehensive national health survey is conducted at five-year intervals (Cayemittes et al. 2007), but its usage and reference appear more widespread among international analysts and donors than among Haitian administrators and clinicians. The Haitian nurses, secretaries, and other professionals who are responsible for collecting data have high stakes in *producing* the data—given that doing so is often tied to their salary and job security—but they have little motivation to understand the data's purpose or ensure their quality, given that the data are generally extracted from their work environment and will not return in any recognizable form. Both Nickerson and Negussie decried this problem, the former describing it in this fashion:

> In my opinion, people's experience with data here is that data has been a necessary evil that's been demanded by an outside funder or someone else, that you need to produce for them to get something back. I've rarely seen people understand it as theirs, they own it, it's their information, it gives them power to know what's going on. It's not about someone else, and it's important, if you want to improve quality of care, you need to know what's going on. So that's the very first step in quality circles: measure things, understand what's going on, then within this environment, within how things work here, what could be done to improve things here, and trying it, and measuring it again. I wouldn't say it's countercultural. It's just historically not a part of how things have been done here, not part of the worldview of how things work. And part of it, one of the currents that we have to swim against is this idea that "we don't own the data." "When people come and measure things here, we never hear what the results are. Someone publishes it, or it's for the purposes of a report for funding somewhere." It's never presented as . . . yours. And I have many, many examples of talking to people about measuring things and having the first response be "Why would we do that, no one's asking for that?"

Negussie describes a situation in which a data collection tool that was also supposed to be a tool to help develop a birthing plan for pregnant woman completely evaded the latter component:

> We have prenatal mobile units, where we go out into the communities and do prenatal care. I was curious about how we actually do them, because of course we get the numbers about how many women were seen, but what does that really mean? What kind of care do they really receive? So I attended a few, and what I noticed that when it

comes to . . . fine, you know, the "What's your name?," "Where do you live?," those things can be perfunctory, but nurses also have to do counseling and education with them with women about where they want to deliver. "Do you know where you want to deliver?" or "Who do you want your baby delivered by?" If the woman says she wants her baby delivered at HUJ, okay, so tell me how are you going to get there. Obviously it's going to take money, it's going to take transportation, it's going to take money once they get there. There needs to be a conversation about that. It needs to be meaningful for the woman, and helping her plan for the birth. What I saw was, "Where are you going to give birth?" The woman says something, the nurse writes it down. "How many months are you into your pregnancy?" She writes it down, basically fills out this birthing plan for the woman, without asking any follow-up question or engaging the woman in a conversation, and then keeps the sheet herself rather than giving that to the woman, because it's now property of the project rather than a tool that helps the women think about or plan for the baby's birth.

Nickerson described the situation this way:

I felt like there's been a misalignment. . . . We're getting paid for the health center to have results, so where's their incentive to do that? The State Department didn't allow us, for instance, to contract with the health facility and then help them achieve these results. We had to hire the people ourselves. From the health center's point of view, it's our program. Why should they care about it? It's nice that we're there, but . . . So we would hire people to produce these widgets. I don't want to continue with that mode. Our goal is that they're functioning to do that. The incentives have to be in line that these are their outcomes, that they're incentivized about those outcomes. If delivering better health isn't enough, than the incentives are in line for them to do that, and if there's a role for us to help them in that, then we're happy to do that. And if there's not, that's okay too.

He added, "I'm all for data. I'm all for data and measuring outcomes. I think the problem is the ownership part. If the system here is going to be self-empowered, it has to own its own data too. And I think that what becomes enculturated is that not only the data is owned by other people, but the outcomes are owned by others."

Konbit Sante as an organization has attempted to remedy this situation with several data collection projects that are directly tied to services within the clinical sites. For example, women who give birth at HUJ's maternity ward are directed to bring their newborns to another building to receive vaccination, but it was unclear what percentage followed these instructions. With Konbit Sante's guidance, the hospital staff developed a system whereby the women were told to bring a slip of paper to the vaccination center, which would then indicate the number of successful referrals. When initial results showed that only 20 percent of the women brought their child for vaccination, the hospital staff had a piece of information that confirmed a serious problem (where before there had only been speculation) and could also serve as a baseline to measure the impact of future interventions.

Conclusion

Both in Haiti and elsewhere the discourse that the country does not have a viable future has gained currency (Beckett 2008). Haitians and international observers use the country's deforestation, overpopulation, chronic political instability, and massive social problems as evidence that Haiti is "finished" and that there is no reasonable hope for the country. Subsumed in this grim prognosis is the prediction that Haiti will never be truly free from international support and assistance. While it is not uncommon, particularly among the most impoverished communities, to hear messages of hope and optimism, these are often expressed in religious idioms, and the messages of resilience and surmounting challenges are expressed in a context where pessimism and discouragement are ubiquitous and at times overwhelming.

One can therefore interpret Konbit Sante's work, as well as the work of other Haitian and international organizations, as a project that is premised on a hopeful forecast of Haiti's health system. While the group does at times measure its accomplishments and successes in quantifiable and immediate outcomes (containers of supplies delivered, health agents hired), it is committed to a style of intervention that cannot always deliver specific or timely results. As Nickerson pointed out to me, some of the organization's earlier interventions and investments took years before producing any results, in part because Haitian staff initially weren't sure if the organization would sustain its presence or close down after a few years of operation, as do so many NGOs in Haiti. Despite high rates of professional emigration, Konbit Sante has been able to maintain and nurture personal relationships and ties for over a decade, and while these relationships and their content would be meaningless if expressed in quantified form, they count among the organization's primary accomplishments.

This has not occurred without challenges or frictions. Any efforts to intervene across steep inequalities will be fraught with unmet expectations, suspicions of misconduct, and questions about why disparities persist despite significant and widespread aid interventions. Rather than seeking out specific individual moral failings or weaknesses, it is important to recognize the broader, structural conditions that lead to aid falling short of its intended results. In the case of medical aid, the tendencies to parse biomedical activities into discrete interventions and use them as a proxy for health—vertical disease eradication campaigns, clinical remedies for preventable conditions—correspond well with the growing demand for rapid and quantifiable results.

These approaches, operating in what Pandolfi and Fassin (2007) refer to as a "state of emergency," are less useful in sketching the contours of what, in the Haitian case, could be described as a "not as dire future." When the staff of Konbit Sante invest in working relationships with Haiti's government, when they continue to support the training of young clinicians who have every reason to leave their country, and when they envision health services informed by locally produced and locally relevant metrics, they gamble on a country and population that many others have wagered against. In playing these unfavorable odds, they join Haitians who, willingly or not, develop the projects that they hope will sustain them into their country's uncertain future.

Notes

1. The term itself is of uncertain provenance but appeared in American speech in the early twentieth century and falls into the category of colloquial expressions (such as *gizmo, doodad*) to indicate indeterminacy, manufactured status, and instrumentality. In the past decade *widget* has also come to refer to a computer or mobile phone application that offers basic information in a continuous manner. I only use the term's earlier meaning in this text.

2. Konbit Sante, "History," accessed August 21, 2014, https://www.konbitsante.org /history.

3. J. Geiger, "Help Needed for School Children in Chantal," We Care to Share Medical-Dental Trips to Chantal, Haiti, April 25, 2015, accessed May 2, 2015 http://chantalhaitimission.wordpress.com/.

4. Clinicians of the World, "2012 Medical Hope for Haiti Medical Trip Report," December 2012, accessed July 15, 2014, http://www.cliniciansoftheworld.org/Dec2012_newsletter.html.

5. First Presbyterian, Ann Arbor, Michigan, "Haiti Medical Mission, accessed July 28, 2014 http://firstpresbyterian.org/mission/international/haiti-medical-mission.

6. It is important to note that these are the components that I most frequently heard mentioned by Konbit Sante's staff and members when describing the organization, although not necessarily in this schematized fashion.

EPILOGUE What Counts in Good Global Health?

VINCANNE ADAMS

If the essays in this volume make us question the assumption that the use of global health metrics will invariably and inevitably lead us to better health outcomes, then we have done our job. We are not alone in calling attention to this problem, but the concerns that now circulate about how we use metrics, what they mean, and what they inadvertently do are concerns that run deep in and through these chapters. What I hope we have shown is not that we should throw the baby out with the bathwater when it comes to using metrics. Metrics can be and often are useful. At the same time, however, it is important to understand how the use of metrics can also interrupt and derail efforts to improve health, no matter what scale we are talking about: local, global, near or far. We need to recognize the limitations of these counting exercises, the use of the kinds of metrics that are being deployed (and to what end), and we need to recognize what other kinds of work metrics do far beyond their rhetorical claims to improving health.

This volume is intended to help us think productively about how metrics create new possibilities and alliances that are changing things in rather dramatic ways for those on the ground, deep in the trenches, trying to achieve, trying to provide, and trying to promote global health. The alliances made possible my metrics are productive in ways that reach far beyond the generation of numbers and facts. Metrics enable certain kinds of medical practices while impeding others. They generate forms of knowledge and certainty about some things even while effacing others. They can authorize new kinds of fiscal investments in health, and new ways of linking market models to health care provision. The metrics used in global health today can even become a lingua franca by which people negotiate global citizenship, sometimes at the expense of national sovereignty. Thus even when metrics efforts end up promoting health, it is important to recognize how the metrics—and not just health seeking, as Nguyen (2010) has shown— are changing the terms and conditions of what constitutes health in relation to governance, politics and markets.

The productivities and effacements that occur through metrics take place at the level of data collection, when it becomes obvious that getting good data (for all the good it can do) can also exact a type of violence of erasure. This can happen when data become a form of political praxis, reflecting a tyranny not just *of numbers* but also *over the numbers*, conditioning what counts and does not count, what can be seen and what needs to be kept invisible. It happens when the numbers are held hostage, not only to advance political goals but also to obtain funding. Violence can happen when the work required to produce metrics undermines good medical practices. Fundamental assumptions about what kinds of evidence should count in global health can figure prominently in determining health resource allocations and the structuring of health in relation to fiscal profits, producing ideals of win-win scenarios where profit making is put in service to health goals. These architectures of global health aid, of finance, and of intervention are today organized around the use of and persistent belief in the power of metrics, but what do we do when the metrics needed to generate profits become more of a distraction from than a source of health benefits? Finally, the large scale reliance on metrics often creates opportunities to standardize our methods of research, but what do we do when we start to treat fidelity to our research method as evidence of success even when this means compromising good care or empirical evidence to the contrary? Just how well these metrics strategies work and how often they don't is not something that can be quantified, but we do know that sometimes the metrics further us toward health goals and sometimes they do not. What is true in any case is that all of the other commitments that come along with the use of metrics is of concern to those of us who are witnessing its outcomes firsthand.

So, given these insights, what hope is there for naming, let alone doing, good global health work in relation to the use of metrics? Do these chapters offer evidence that metrics are fallible but still of use? Or do they suggest that the metrics we have deployed are inherently, epistemologically flawed? If so, what are the alternatives to metrical forms of truth? To answer this, I want to turn, in this last instance, to the possibility of engaging in another kind of conversation about the methods we use in global health, and to other ways of thinking about metrics.

Social science critiques make a positive contribution by showing how things work and don't work not just in theory but in practice, and by sometimes serving as a witness to and voice for those who are not able to speak back to the overarching demands for certain forms of evidence that are placed on them. At the same time, we should heed the advice of Fletcher Linder (2012), and avoid adopting the Neitzchean notion of "slave ethics" in our critical witnessing. Slave ethics define the position of subordination to the master's ethics, but also reinforce the latter by way of critique. No one explains the problem of power better than those who have none. If we are to make inroads that will not only change the model of our global health engagements but also the health of those we hope to help, he suggests a form of critically applied anthropology. To me, this sort of engagement means not simply pointing out the failures of metrics, or even the way that the success of metrics in global health work against us, and sometimes against health. Rather, we need to explore new ways of talking about metrics that undo their claims on certainty, on standardization and truth, and simultaneously pursue new models that may be worth pursuing.

To begin with, it is useful to acknowledge the many anthropologists and social scientists who are working in the trenches of public health and epidemiology, trying to wrestle with the challenges of incorporating ethnographic evidence into RCT research and intervention endeavors. Studies from sociology, public health, anthropology, and other fields suggest creative integration of the critical methods of social science in RCT research (Colvin 2014; Rapkin and Trickett 2005; Smith-Morris et al. 2014). These studies show us that when ethnographic data are incorporated into the design of research, even in the case of RCT research, the back and forth between the different kinds of data they produce can be productive not only for improving care practices but also in accounting for what factors ultimately work to improve health outcomes. There is often a hopeful engagement in these works for futures that can live within the regimes of RCTs. Whether or not hopefulness is warranted is something the chapters in this volume suggest should remain an open question.

Similar forms of both optimism and skepticism are aroused in efforts to use ethnography to study the sociologies of metrics, documenting the cocreation of regimes of epidemiology in global health. As rubrics for data collection become the organizing principles for treatment or therapy, these rubrics form new kinds of social beings, social relationships, and political identities (Crane 2013; Lorway and Khan 2014; Nguyen 2010). Scientific knowledge is cocreated alongside data in these efforts, but so too are social realities that subjects are asked to inhabit, and all of these should be recognized as outcomes that matter, for better or worse, in relation to health. Again these are, in some ways, exactly the sorts of practices this volume has questioned and the kinds of practices that can be worrisome.

Beyond these optimistic engagements, there are assurances that creative forms of resistance to narrow uses of statistical and RCT metrics are out there. Michael Fischer (2013), for instance, describes disruptions to RCT determinism among those who suffer from "orphan diseases." Because the number of people who suffer from these diseases is frequently not high enough to constitute a basis for robust clinical trials, these patients have begun to make arguments for quantification strategies using an "n of 1," such that their own bodies become the site for the production of metrics. This tactic in some ways combines the radical possibility of using subjective experience, even while capitulating to the demand for quantification that experimental standards demand. Similarly researchers in the HIV/AIDS prevention world are often confronted with the need to move the goalposts of RCT designs, for instance calling into question the use of blind RCT methods[1]—a move that reflects both the inadequacy of the model and the dream of inventing a new and improved version of it. Finally, the "quantified self" movement, in which subjects devote considerable time and energy mapping their health vis-à-vis its quantifiable patterns, might be seen as part of this trend toward an "n of 1" as well.[2] Here the ways quantification behaviors map onto market strategies, even while in some sense deflecting them as a form of resistance, is intriguing. The use of metrics here suggests an almost satirical use in ways that bolster notions of objectivity while collapsing truth onto the site of the singular subject.

Another new trend that suggests a subtle form of resistance within capitulation to the metrics is the growth of research protocols that use a feedback loop between protocol modifications and follow-up of those subjects whose outcomes are seen as failures. Thus researchers who track the reasons people fall out of clinical trials or whose results are negative, for instance, can be studied for evidence of potential sites for improvement upon, modification of, or the need for new designs for the study. Consider, for instance, a study that interrogates why vaccines are rejected by villagers and uses this information to remap interventions that address these failures rather than simply treating them as evidence that vaccine programs fail. In some ways the RCT is celebrated because of this sense of its flexibility. Surely, by the time this volume is published there will be a whole new generation of global health scholars who have reinvented the RCT so that they can capture any imagined health outcome. How these uses of the RCT both deconstruct familiar notions of standardization and scalability, while also working with the technique of experimentalism, pose interesting possibilities for new models of evidence-based global health.

One of the overarching insights of this volume might be to suggest that this revisionist strategy to continually move the goalposts of the RCT until we get it right is like a game of logarithmically diminishing returns — a situation in which, because of the form RCT knowledge takes, efforts may get closer and closer to closing the gap, but it will never actually succeed because we must continually reinvent the same unsuccessful models for intervention and data collection. Again the strategy of "research as intervention" proliferates here, even to the point of an involution of its prodigious production of data. On the other hand, it is useful to think about how this technique undermines, even while reinforcing, traditional forms of RCT epistemology so that they still, ironically, can be used to deliver important health interventions.

There are a growing number of cases that describe how efforts to do pharmaceutical RCT research get shut down or modified by political opposition, forcing researchers to shift their focus and do work that is perhaps, in the end, more suitable to the on-the-ground needs of the community (Geissler 2011; Yamey 2011). It might be useful to think about how these radical alternatives and resistances could be used in efforts to sustain program funding by using this kind of data. In all, these efforts provide indications that traditional RCT models are under revision and that data emerging from and about ethnographically complex contexts remain vital to doing good global health work.

Finally, I point to the ongoing work of global health organizations like Partners in Health, whose human rights approach to health care offers alternatives to experimentalist models advanced by the large global health institutions. I also call attention to efforts to identify good quality global health research in ways that prioritize the tools and skills of ethnography, as against those of RCT data collecting. Pigg (2013) reminds us of the generative power of tapping into traditional methods of ethnographic participant observation that involved "sitting" as an imperative for critical reflection that can inform our sense of "doing." Elsewhere my colleagues and I have proposed rethinking the paradigm of global health research (Adams et al. 2014, forthcoming). Calling our method "slow research" and proposing "alternative forms of accounting," we point to the advantages of keeping our efforts local, pluralizing our strategies so they can be tailored to specific sites, scaling across rather than scaling up as forms of dynamic engagement with differences, institutional practices on the ground, and the need for flexibility. All of these efforts invite a rethinking of what we mean by *evidence* in our efforts to create accountability. They pose alternatives to the models of comprehensive dynamic trial designs found in the clinical trials research, reminding us that far beyond the world of RCTs and Millennium Development Goals–style counting exercises (whether the Global Burden of Disease index or the Disability-Adjusted Life Years) there is crucial information that is necessary for global health. Still, alternative engagements that unseat tendencies toward the tyranny of numbers are plentiful but woefully underutilized in global health today. My hope, shared by others in this volume, is that this book will address this underutilization by making it clear that the kinds of evidence found throughout these pages are, in fact, foundational to being able to establish a positive agenda in global health.

Notes

1. See the discussion of this in relation to development of drugs at U.S. House of Representatives, Energy and Commerce Committee, "Energy and Commerce Cures," accessed February 18, 2015, http://energycommerce.house.gov/cures.

2. Dana Greenfield, a graduate student in the MD/PhD program at UCSF, explores this in her doctoral dissertation.

REFERENCES

AbouZahr, Carla. 2011. "New Estimates of Maternal Mortality and How to Interpret Them: Choice or Confusion?" *Reproductive Health Matters* 19(37): 117–28.

Abraham, John, and Rachel Ballinger. 2012. "The Neoliberal State, Industry Interests, and the Ideological Penetration of Scientific Knowledge: Deconstructing the Redefinition of Carcinogens in Pharmaceuticals." *Science, Technology and Human Values* 37: 443–77.

Adams, Vincanne. 2002. "Randomized Controlled Crime: Postcolonial Sciences in Alternative Medicine Research." *Social Studies of Science* 32(5/6): 659–90.

———. 2005. "Saving Tibet? An Inquiry into Modernity, Lies, Truths, and Belief." *Medical Anthropology* 24(1): 71–110.

———. 2012. "The Other Road to Serfdom: Recovery by the Market and the Affect Economy in New Orleans." *Public Culture* 24(1): 185–216.

———. 2013a. "Evidence Based Global Public Health: Subjects, Profits, Erasures." In J. Biehl and A. Petryna, eds., *When People Come First*, 54–90. Princeton: Princeton University Press.

———. 2013b. *Markets of Sorrow, Labors of Faith: New Orleans in the Wake of Katrina.* Durham: Duke University Press.

Adams, Vincanne, et al. 2005. "The Challenge of Cross-cultural Clinical Trials Research: Case Report from the Tibetan Autonomous Region, People's Republic of China." *Medical Anthropology Quarterly* 19(3): 267–89.

Adams, Vincanne, Nancy J. Burke, and Ian Whitmarsh. 2014. "Slow Research: Thoughts for a Movement in Global Health." *Medical Anthropology* 33(3): 179–97.

Adams, Vincanne, Sienna R. Craig, and Arlene Samen. Forthcoming. "Alternative Accounting in Maternal and Infant Health." *Global Public Health.*

Adams, Vincanne, M. Murphy, and A. Clarke. 2009. "Anticipation: Technoscience, Life, Affect, Temporality." *Subjectivity* 28(1): 246–65.

Allotey, P., D. Reidpath, A. Kouame, and R. Cummins. 2003. "The DALY, Context and

Determinants of the Severity of Disease: An Exploratory Comparison of Paraplegia in Australia and Cameroon." *Social Science and Medicine* 57(5): 949–58.

Anand, Sudhir, and Kara Hanson. 1997. "Disability Adjusted Life Years: A Critical Review." *Journal of Health Economics* 16: 685–702.

Anderson, Warwick. 2006. *Colonial Pathologies: American Tropical Medicine, Race and Hygiene in the Philippines*. Durham: Duke University Press.

Armstrong, David. 1995. "The Rise of Surveillance Medicine." *Sociology of Health & Illness* 17(3): 393–404.

Arnesen, Trude, and Lydia Kapiriri. 2004. "Can the Value Choices in DALYs Influence Global Priority Setting?" *Health Policy* 70: 137–49.

Arnesen, Trude, and Erik Nord. 1999. "The Value of DALY Life: Problems with Ethics and Validity of Disability Adjusted Life Years." *BMJ* 319(7222): 1423–25.

Arzac, Enrique R. 1986. "Do Your Business Units Create Shareholder Value?" *Harvard Business Review* (Jan.–Feb.): 121–26.

Bajracharya, Ashish, Ben Bellows, and Antonia Dingle. 2013. "Evaluation of a Voucher Programme in Reducing Inequities in Maternal Health Utilisation in Cambodia: A Quasi-experimental Study." *Lancet* 381(S12). http://www.thelancet.com/journals/lancet/article/PIIS0140-6736(13)61266-0/abstract.

Banerjee, A., A. Hollis, and T. Pogge. 2013. "The Health Impact Fund: Incentives for Improving Access to Medicines. *Lancet* 375: 166–69.

Banerjee, Abhijit, and Esther Duflo. 2011 *Poor Economics: A Radical Rethinking of the Way to Fight Global Poverty*. New York: Public Affairs.

Banerji, D., and Stig Anderson. 1963. "A Sociological Study of Awareness of Symptoms among Persons with Pulmonary Tuberculosis." *Bulletin of the World Health Organization* 29(5): 665–83.

Bartelson, Jens. 2006. "The Concept of Sovereignty Revisited." *European Journal of International Law* 17(2): 463–74.

Basu, Sanjay. 2011. "Corporate Links of Global Health Foundations May Conflict with Philanthropic Interests." *e! Science News*, April 12. Accessed November 18, 2013. http://esciencenews.com/articles/2011/04/12/corporate.links.global.health.foundations.may.conflict.with.philanthropic.interest.

————. 2012. "Blah Blah Blah: A Jaded Calculation of the Rhetoric-to Results Ratio in Public Health." Global Health Hub. September 13. http://www.globalhealthhub.org/2012/09/13/rhetoric/.

Batha, Emma. 2011. "Haiti Loses Its Doctors and Nurses to Aid Groups." Alertnet. January 14. http://www.trust.org/alertnet/news/haiti-loses-doctors-and-nurses-to-aid-groups-report/.

Becker, Deborah R., et al. 2006. "What Predicts Supported Employment Program Outcomes?" *Community Mental Health Journal* 42(3): 303–13.

Becker, D. R., et al. 2001. "Fidelity of Supported Employment Programs and Employment Outcomes." *Psychiatric Services* 52(6): 834–36.

Becker, Anne, Anjali Motgi, Jonathan Wiegel, Giuseppe Raviola, Salmaan Keshavjee, and Arthur Kleinman. 2013. "The Unique Challenges of Mental Health and MDRTB: Critical Perspectives on Metrics of Diseases." In P. Farmer, J. Y. Kim,

A. Kleinman, and M. Basilico, eds., *Reimagining Global Health: An Introduction*, 212–44. Berkeley: University of California Press.

Beckett, Gregory. 2008. "The End of Haiti: History under Conditions of Impossibility." PhD diss., University of Chicago.

Begg, C. B., et al. 1996. "Improving the Quality of Reporting of Randomized Controlled Trials: The CONSORT statement." *Journal of the American Medical Association* 276: 637–39.

Biehl, Joao. 2008. "Drugs for All: The Future of Global AIDS Treatment." *Medical Anthropology* 27(2): 1–7.

———. 2013. "The Judicialization of Biopolitics: Claiming the Right to Pharmaceuticals in Brazilian Courts." *American Ethnologist* 240(3): 419–36.

Biehl, Joao, and Adriana Petryna, eds. 2013. *When People Come First: Critical Studies in Global Health*. Princeton: Princeton University Press.

Bill and Melinda Gates Foundation. 2013. "Annual Letter 2013." Accessed January 21, 2014. http://www.gatesfoundation.org/Who-We-Are/Resources-and-Media/Annual-Letters-List/Annual-Letter-2013.

———. 2014a. "Foundation Fact Sheet." Accessed June 26, 2014. http://www.gatesfoundation.org/Who-We-Are/General-Information/Foundation-Factsheet.

———. 2014b. "What We Do: Malaria, Strategy Overview." Accessed April 4, 2014. http://www.gatesfoundation.org/What-We-Do/Global-Health/Malaria.

Birn, Anne-Emanuelle. 2005. "Gates's Grandest Challenge: Transcending Technology as Public Health Ideology." *Lancet*, March 11. http://image.thelancet.com/extras/04art6429web.pdf.

———. 2014. "Philanthrocapitalism, Past and Present: The Rockefeller Foundation, the Gates Foundation and the Setting(s) of the International/Global Health Agenda." *Hypothesis* 12(1): 1–27.

Birn, Anne-Emanuelle, Yogan Pillay, and Timothy H. Holtz. 2009. *Textbook of International Health: Global Health in a Dynamic World*. 3rd ed. New York: Oxford University Press.

Biruk, Crystal. 2012. "Seeing Like a Research Project: Producing 'High Quality Data' in AIDS Research in Malawi." *Medical Anthropology* 31(4): 347–66.

Bishai, David, Karampreet Sachathep, and Amnesty E. LeFevre. 2013. "Determining the Cost-Effectiveness of Managing Acute Diarrhea through Social Franchising of ORASEL: A Randomized Controlled Trial." *Lancet* 381(s17). http://www.thelancet.com/journals/lancet/article/PIIS0140-6736(13)61271-4/abstract.

Bond, G. R., et al. 2001. Dimensions of Supported Employment: Factor Structure of the IPS Fidelity Scale. *Journal of Mental Health* 10(4): 383–93.

Bond, Gary R 2004. Supported Employment: Evidence for an Evidence-based Practice. *Psychiatric Rehabilitation Journal* 27(4): 345.

Bond, G. R., R. E. Drake, and D. R. Becker. 2008a. "An Update on Randomized Controlled Trials of Evidence-based Supported Employment." *Psychiatric Rehabilitation Journal* 31(4): 280–90.

Bond, G. R., R. E. Drake, and D. R. Becker. 2008b. "Fidelity of Supported Employment: Lessons Learned from the National." *Psychiatric Rehabilitation Journal* 31(4): 300–305.

Bordes, Ary. 1992. *Médecine et Sante Publique en Haïti: Période de l'Occupation américaine, 1915–1934*. Port-au-Prince: Henri Deschamps.

———. 1997. *La Sante de la Republique, 1934–1957*. Port-au-Prince: Henri Deschamps.

Bornstein, Erica. 2005. *The Spirit of Development: Protestant NGOs, Morality and Economics in Zimbabwe*. London: Routledge.

Bose, Sugata. 1997. "Instruments and Idioms of Colonial and National Development: India's Historical Experience in Comparative Perspective." In F. Cooper and R. Packard, eds., *International Development and the Social Sciences*, 45–63. Berkeley: University of California Press.

Bowker, Geoffrey C., and Susan Leigh Star. 1999. *Sorting Things Out*. Cambridge, MA: MIT Press.

Bowman, Candice C., et al. 2008. Measuring Persistence of Implementation: QUERI Series. *Implementation Science* 3(1): 21.

Brave Heart, M. Y. H. 2004. "The Historical Trauma Response among Natives and Its Relationship to Substance Abuse: A Lakota Illustration." In E. Nebelkopf and M. Phillips, eds., *Healing and Mental Health for Native Americans: Speaking in Red*, 7–18. Walnut Creek, CA: Alta Mira Press.

Brenneis, Don. 2010. "Regimes of Recognition: Metrics, Models and 'Academic Charisma.'" Paper presented at the Department of Sociology, University of Hong Kong May 24.

Brown, E. Richard. 1976. "Public Health in Imperialism: Early Rockefeller Programs at Home and Abroad." *American Journal of Public Health* 66(9): 897–903.

———. 1979. *Rockefeller Medicine Men: Medicine and Capitalism in America*. Berkeley: University of California Press.

Brown, Theodore M., Marcos Cueto, and Elizabeth Fee. 2006. "The World Health Organization and the Transition from 'International' to 'Global' Public Health." *American Journal of Public Health* 96(1): 62–72.

Bui, Linh N., et al. 2013. "Risk Factors of Burden of Disease: A Comparative Assessment Study for Evidence-based Health Policy Making in Vietnam." *Lancet* 381(s23). http://www.thelancet.com/journals/lancet/article/PIIS0140-6736(13)61277-5/abstract.

Buse, Kent, and Sara Hawkes. 2015. "Health in the Sustainable Development Goals: Ready for a Paradigm Shift?" *Globalization and Health* 11:13. doi:10.1186/s12992-015-0098-8.

Buse, K., and G. Walt. 1997. "An Unruly Mélange? Coordinating External Resources to the Health Sector: A Review." *Social Science and Medicine* 45(3): 449–63.

Butt, Leslie. 2002. "The Suffering Stranger: Medical Anthropology and International Morality." *Medical Anthropology* 21: 1–24.

Canguilhem, Georges. 1991. *The Normal and the Pathological*. New York: Zone Books.

Carpenter, C. 1994. "The Experience of Spinal Cord Injury: The Individual's Perspective — Implications for Rehabilitation." *Physical Therapy* 74: 614–29.

Cassini, Alessandro, et al. 2013. "Improving the Usability and Communication of Burden of Disease Methods and Outputs: The Experience of the Burden of Communicable Diseases in Europe Software Toolkit," *Lancet* 381(S27). http://www.the lancet.com/journals/lancet/article/PIIS0140-6736(13)61281-7/abstract.

Cattelino, Jessica. 2008. *High Stakes: Florida Seminole Gaming and Sovereignty.* Durham: Duke University Press.

Cayemittes, Michel, Marie Florence Placide, Soumaïla Mariko, Bernard Barrère, Blaise Sévère, and Canez Alexandre. 2007. *Enquête Mortalité, Morbidité et Utilisation des Services, Haïti 2005–2006.* Calverton, MD: Ministère de la Santé Publique et de la Population, Institut Haïtien de l'Enfance and Macro International.

Chandler, David. 2001. "The Road to Military Humanitarianism: How the Human Rights NGOs Shaped a New Humanitarian Agenda." *Human Rights Quarterly* 23(3): 678–700.

Chang, L. W., et al. 2010. "Developing WHO Guidelines with Pragmatic, Structured, Evidence-based Processes: A Case Study." *Global Public Health: An International Journal for Research, Policy and Practice* 5(4): 395–412.

Chapin, Martha H., and Donald G. Kewman. 2001. "Factors Affecting Employment Following Spinal Cord Injury: A Qualitative Study." *Rehabilitation Psychology* 46(4): 400–416.

Chorev, Nitsan. 2012. *The World Health Organization between North and South.* Ithaca: Cornell University Press.

Closser, Svea. 2010. *Chasing Polio in Pakistan: Why the World's Largest Health Initiative May Fail.* Nashville: Vanderbilt University Press.

Cohen, Jon. 2012. "A Controversial Close-up of Humanity's Health." *Science* 338(6113): 1414–16.

Cohen, Lawrence. 2004. "Operability: Surgery at the Margin of the State." In Veena Das and Deborah Poole, eds., *Anthropology in the Margins of the State*, 165–90. Santa Fe: SAR Press.

Colvin, Christopher J. 2014. "Anthropologies in and of Evidence Making in Global Health Research and Policy." *Medical Anthropology* doi: 10.1080/01459740.2014. 063196 (online version).

Comaroff, Jean, and John Comaroff. 2001. "Millennial Capitalism: First Thoughts on a Second Coming." In Jean Comaroff and John Comaroff, eds., *Millennial Capitalism and the Culture of Neoliberalism*, 1–56. Durham: Duke University Press.

Cooper, Fred. 1997. "Modernizing Bureaucrats, Backward Africans, and the Development Concept." In F. Cooper and R. Packard, eds., *International Development and the Social Sciences: Essays on the History and Politics of Knowledge.* Berkeley: University of California Press.

Cooper, Frederick, and Randall Packard, eds. 1997. *International Development and the Social Sciences: Essays on the History and Politics of Knowledge.* Berkeley: University of California Press.

Cooper, Melinda. 2008. *Life as Surplus: Biotechnology and Capitalism in the Neoliberal Era.* Seattle: University of Washington Press.

Craddock, Susan. 2012. "Drug Partnerships and Global Practices." *Health and Place* 18: 481–89.

Crane, Johanna. 2010a. "Adverse Events and Placebo Effects: African Scientists, HIV, and Ethics in the 'Global Health Sciences.'" *Social Studies of Science* 40(6): 843–70.

———. 2010b. "Unequal 'Partners': AIDS, Academia, and the Rise of Global Health." *Behemoth* 3(3): 78–97.

———. 2013. *Scrambling for Africa: AIDS, Expertise and the Rise of American Global Health Science*. Ithaca: Cornell University Press.

Crump, Thomas. 1990. *The Anthropology of Numbers*. Cambridge: Cambridge University Press.

Daly, Jeanne. 2005. *Evidence-based Medicine and the Search for a Science of Clinical Care*. Berkeley: University of California Press.

Das, Veena. 1999. "Public Good, Ethics, and Everyday Life: Beyond the Boundaries of Bioethics." *Daedalus* 128(4): 99–133.

Daston, Lorraine J., and Peter Galison. 2010. *Objectivity*. New York: Zone Books.

Davis, Georgia, and Mark Nichter. 2015. "The Lyme Wars: The Effects of Bio-communicability, Gender, and Epistemic Politics on Health Activation and Lyme Science." In Carolyn Smith-Morris, ed., *Diagnostic Controversy: Social Context at the Edge of Medical Certainty*. New York: Routledge.

Deaton, Angus. 2010. "Instruments, Randomization, and Learning about Development." *Journal of Economic Literature* 48(2): 424–55.

Deloria, Vine, Jr., and Clifford M. Lytle. 1984. *The Nations Within: The Past and Future of American Indian Sovereignty*. Austin: University of Texas Press.

Demakis, John G., et al. 2000. "Quality Enhancement Research Initiative (QUERI): A Collaboration between Research and Clinical Practice." *Medical Care* 38(6): 117–125, QUERI Supplement.

Derman, Emanuel. 2004. *My Life as a Quant: Reflections on Physics and Finance*. Hoboken, NJ: John Wiley & Sons.

De Waal, A. 1997. *Famine Crimes: Politics and the Disaster Relief Industry in Africa*. Bloomington: Indiana University Press.

Dubois, Carl-Ardy, France Brunelle, and Carine Rousseau. 2007. *Analyses et Projection: Recensement des Ressources Humaines en Santé en Haïti. Technical Report*. Montréal: Project PARC, Unité de Santé Internationale, Université de Montréal.

Duflo, Esther, Rachel Glennerster, and Michael Kremer. 2008. "Using Randomization in Development Economics Research: A Toolkit." In T. Paul Schultz and John Strauss, eds., *Handbook of Development Economics*, vol. 4, 3895–962. Oxford: Elsevier.

Dumit, Joe. 2012. *Drugs for Life: How Pharmaceutical Companies Define Our Health*. Durham: Duke University Press.

Edlow, J. A., et al. 2013. "Diagnosis of Acute Neurological Emergencies in Pregnant and Post-partum Women." *Lancet Neurology* 12(2): 175–85.

Erikson, Susan L. 2008. "Getting Political: Fighting Smarter for Global Health." *Lancet* 371(9620): 1229–30.

———. 2011. "Global Ethnography: Problems of Theory and Method." In

Carole C. H. Browner and Carolyn F. Sargent, eds., *Globalization, Reproduction, and the State*, 23–37. Durham: Duke University Press.

———. 2012. "Global Health Business: The Production and Performativity of Statistics in Sierra Leone and Germany." In "Enumeration, Identity, and Health." Special issue of *Medical Anthropology* 32(4): 367–84.

———. 2015a. "Global Health Indicators and Maternal Health Futures: The Case of Intrauterine Growth Restriction." *Global Public Health*, forthcoming.

———. 2015b. "Secrets from Whom? Following the Money in Global Health Finance. *Current Anthropology*, forthcoming.

Escobar, Arturo. 1994. *Encountering Development: The Making and Unmaking of the Third World*. Princeton: Princeton University Press.

———. 2011(1994). *Encountering Development: The Making and Unmaking of the Third World*. Princeton: Princeton University Press.

Farley, John. 2003. *To Cast Out Disease: A History of the International Health Division of the Rockefeller Foundation (1913–1951)*. Oxford: Oxford University Press.

———. 2006. *To Cast Out Disease: A History of the International Health Division of the Rockefeller Foundation, 1913–1951*. Oxford: Oxford University Press.

Farmer, Paul. 2001. *Infections and Inequalities: The Modern Plagues*. Berkeley: University of California Press.

Farmer, Paul, Jim Yong Kim, Arthur Kleinman, and Matthew Basilico, eds. 2013. *Reimagining Global Health: An Introduction*. Berkeley: University of California Press.

Fassin, Didier. 2012. *Humanitarian Reason: A Moral History of the Present*. Berkeley: University of California Press.

Feierman, Steven. 2010. "When Physicians Meet: Local Knowledge and Global Public Goods." In W. Geissler and S. Molyneux, eds., *The Ethnography of Medical Research in Africa*. New York: Berghahn.

Ferguson, James. 1994. *The Anti-Politics Machine: "Development," Depoliticization, and Bureaucratic Power in Lesotho*. Rev. ed. Minneapolis: University of Minnesota Press.

———. 2006. *Global Shadows: Africa in the Neoliberal World Order*. Durham: Duke University Press.

Finnemore, Martha. 1997. "Redefining Development at the World Bank." In F. Cooper and R. Packard, eds., *International Development and the Social Sciences*, 203–27. Berkeley: University of California Press.

Fioramonti, Lorenzo. 2014. *How Numbers Rule the World: The Use and Abuse of Statistics in Global Politics*. New York: Zed Books.

Fischer, Michael. 2013. "Conclusion." In J. Biehl and A. Petryna, eds., *When People Come First: Critical Studies in Global Health*. Princeton: Princeton University Press.

Floridi, Maurizo, Mamour Ngalane, and Mamadou Lamine Thiam. 2008. *Cartographie des acteurs non étatiques au Sénégal*. Recruited by the European Cabinet Consultants Organization. Dakar, Senegal.

Foley, Ellen. 2009. *Your Pocket Is What Cures You: The Politics of Health in Senegal*. New Brunswick, NJ: Rutgers University Press.

Foucault, Michel. 1977. *Discipline and Punish*. Trans. Alan Sheridan. New York: Vintage Books.

———. 1994. "The Subject and Power." In James D. Faubion, ed., Robert Hurley et al., trans., *Power: Essential Works of Foucault 1954–1984*, 326–48. New York: New Press.

———. 2000. *Power: Essential Works of Michel Foucault 1954–1984*. Vol. 3. Ed. J. Faubion. Trans. R. Hurley et al. London: Allen Lane.

———. 2003. *"Society Must Be Defended": Lectures at the College de France, 1975–1976*. Trans. David Macey. New York: Picador.

———. 2007. *Security, Territory, Population: Lectures at the College de France 1977–1978*. Ed. Michel Senellart. Trans. Graham Burchell. New York: Picador.

———. 2008. *The Birth of Biopolitics*. Ed. Michel Senellart. Trans. Graham Burchell. New York: Picador.

Freire, P. 1970. *Pedagogy of the Oppressed*. New York: Herder and Herder.

Freschi, Laura, and Alanna Shaikh. 2011. "Gates: A Benevolent Dictator for Public Health?" *Alliance* 16(3): 36–37.

Frichner, Tonya Gonnella. 2010. "The Indian Child Welfare Act: A National Law Controlling the Welfare of Indigenous Children." American Indian Law Alliance. https://www.childwelfare.gov/systemwide/courts/icwa.cfm.

Friedman, Milton. 1970. "The Social Responsibility of Business Is to Increase Its Profits." *The New York Times Magazine*, September 13.

Gates, Bill. 2013. "My Annual Letter: How We Measure Impact to Improve Lives." Bill and Melinda Gates Foundation. January 29. http://www.gatesnotes.com/About-Bill-Gates/2013-Annual-Letter.

Gates, Melinda. 2013. "Measuring, Contraception and Investing in Families' Futures." Bill and Melinda Gates Foundation. January 29. http://www.gatesfoundation.org/Who-We-Are/Resources-and-Media/Annual-Letters-List/Annual-Letter-2013.

Gaudillière, Jean Paul. 2015. "De la santé publique internationale à la santé globale: L'OMS, la Banque Mondiale et le gouvernement des thérapies chimiques." In D. Pestre, ed. *Le gouvernement des sciences à l'échelle globale*, 65–96. Paris: La Découverte, 2015.

Geissler, P. Wenzel. 2011. "Introduction: Studying Trial Communities. Anthropological and Historical Inquiries into Ethos, Politics and Economy of Medical Research in Africa." In P. Wenzel Geissler and Catherine Molyneux, eds., *Evidence, Ethos and Experiment: The Anthropology and History of Medical Research in Africa*, 1–28. Oxford: Berghahn Books.

Geissler, P. Wenzel, Ann Kelly, Babatunde Imoukhuede, and Robert Pool. 2008. "'He Is Kike a Brother, I Can Even Give Him Some Blood'—Relational Ethics and Material Exchanges in a Malaria Vaccine 'Trial Community' in the Gambia." *Social Science and Medicine* 67: 696–707.

Geissler, P. Wenzel, and Catherine Molyneux. 2011. *Evidence, Ethos and Experiment: The Anthropology and History of Medical Research in Africa*. New York: Berghahn Books.

Geltzer, Anna. 2009. "When the Standards Aren't Standard: Evidence-based Medicine in the Russian Context." *Social Science and Medicine* 68: 526–32.

GHME Conference Organizing Committee. 2011. "Shared Innovations in Measurement and Evaluation. *Lancet.* doi: 10.1016/S0140-6736(11)60169-4, online.

Global Fund to Fight AIDS, Tuberculosis and Malaria. 2012. *Audit of Global Fund to the Republic of Senegal, GF-OIG-11-007.* Dakar: Office of the Inspector General.

————. 2013. *Grant Performance Report: Senegal, SNG-M-PNLP.* Dakar: Office of the Inspector General. Online. Accessed October 25, 2013.

Global Health Investment Fund. 2014. "An Audience with Bill Gates." Accessed August 31, 2014. http://ghif.com/?s=an+audience+with+bill+gates.

Global Health Watch. 2011. "Conflicts of Interest within Philanthrocapitalism." Accessed June 19, 2013. http://www.ghwatch.org/sites/www.ghwatch.org/files/D3_0.pdf.

Gold, Marthe R., David Stevenson, and Dennis G. Fryback. 2002. "HALYs and QALYs and DALYs, Oh My: Similarities and Differences in Summary Measures of Population Health." *Annual Review of Public Health* 23: 115–34.

Good, Byron. 1994. "Medical Anthropology and the Problem of Belief." In *Medicine, Rationality, and Experience,* 1–24. Cambridge: Cambridge University Press.

Good, Charles M. 1991. "Pioneer Medical Missions in Colonial Africa." *Social Science and Medicine* 32(1): 1–10.

Gordon, Myron J., and Eli Shapiro. 1956. "Capital Equipment Analysis: The Required Rate of Profit." *Management Science* 3(1): 102–10.

Gould, Stephen. J. 1996. *The Mismeasure of Man.* New York: Norton.

Govindarajan, Vijay. 2012. "A Reverse-Innovation Playbook." *Strategic Direction* 28(9). Accessed June 12, 2015. http://www.emeraldinsight.com/doi/abs/10.1108/sd.2012.05628iaa.008?journalCode=sd.

Govindarajan, Vijay, and Chris Trimble. 2012. "Reverse Innovation: A Global Growth Strategy That Could Pre-empt Disruption at Home." *Strategy & Leadership* 40(5): 5–11.

Greene, Jeremy. 2008. *Prescribing by Numbers: Drugs and the Definition of Disease.* Baltimore: Johns Hopkins University Press.

————. 2011. "Making Medicines Essential: The Evolving Role of Pharmaceuticals in Global Health." *Biosocieties* 6: 10–33.

Guyer, Jane. 2004. *Marginal Gains: Monetary Transactions in Atlantic.* Chicago: University of Chicago Press.

Hacking, Ian. 1990. *The Taming of Chance.* Cambridge: Cambridge University Press.

Hammell, K. Whalley. 2007. "Experience of Rehabilitation Following Spinal Cord Injury: A Meta-synthesis of Qualitative Findings." *Spinal Cord* 45: 260–74.

Harding, Sandra. 1998. *Is Science Multicultural? Postcolonialisms, Feminisms, and Epistemologies.* Bloomington: Indiana University Press.

Hardt, Michael, and Antonio Negri. 2001. *Empire.* Cambridge: Harvard University Press.

Harper, Ian. 2006. "Anthroplogy, DOTS and Understanding tuberculosis control in Nepal." *Journal of Biosocial Science* 38: 57–67.

Haskell, Thomas. 1985. "Capitalism and the Origins of the Humanitarian Sensibility, Part 2." *American Historical Review* 90(3): 547–66.

Hefferan, Tara. 2007. *Twinning Faith and Development: Catholic Parish Partnership in the U.S. and Haiti.* West Hartford, CT: Kumarian Press.

Hesperian Health Guides. 2013. "Impact." Hesperian Health Guides. April 22. Accessed April 23, 2013. http://hesperian.org/about/impact/.

Hirimuthugoda, Lasantha K., et al. 2013. "Experimental Design: Impact of an Intervention to Improve Clinic Attendance of Patients with Non-communicable Diseases through Telephone Follow-up." *Lancet* 381(s63). http://www.thelancet.com/journals/lancet/article/PIIS0140-6736(13)61317-3/abstract.

Hodžić, Saida. 2013. "Ascertaining Deadly Harms: Aesthetics and Politics of Global Evidence." *Cultural Anthropology* 28(1): 86–109.

Hogan, Margaret C., et al. 2010. "Maternal Mortality for 181 Countries, 1980–2008: A Systematic Analysis of Progress towards Millennium Development Goal 5." *Lancet* 375: 1609–23.

Hollis, Aidan, and Thomas Pogge. 2008. "The Health Impact Fund: Making New Medicines Accessible for All: A Report of Incentives for Global Health." New Haven: Incentives for Global Health.

Holmes, Dave, Stuart J. Murray, Amelie Perron, and Genevieve Rail. 2006. "Deconstructing the Evidence-based Discourse in Health Sciences: Truth, Power and Fascism." *International Journal of Evidence-Based Healthcare* 4(3): 180–86.

Holmes, Seth. 2013. *Fresh Fruit, Broken Bodies.* Berkeley: University of California Press.

Horton, Richard. 2010. "Maternal Mortality: Surprise, Hope, and Urgent Action." *Lancet* 375(9726): 1581–82.

———. 2013. "Metrics for What?" *Lancet* 381: s1–s2, June 17. doi:10.1016/S0140-6736(13): 61256–58.

Horstmann, Fallon, and Alan D. Lopez. 2013. "Strengthening Vital Registration and Vital Statistics: A Standard-based Toolkit." *Lancet* 381(s64). http://www.thelancet.com/journals/lancet/article/PIIS0140-6736(13)61318-5/fulltext.

Howland, Douglas, and Luise White. 2009. "Introduction: Sovereignty and the Study of States." In D. Howland and L. White, eds., *The State of Sovereignty: Territories, Laws, Populations,* 1–18. Bloomington: Indiana University Press.

Huhndorf, Roy, and Shari M. Huhndorf. 2011. "Alaska Native Politics since the Alaska Native Claims Settlement Act." *South Atlantic Quarterly* 110(2): 385–401.

Immelt, Jeffrey R., Vijay Govindarajan, and Chris Trimble. 2009 "How GE Is Disrupting Itself." *Harvard Business Review* 87(10): 56–65.

Institute for Health Metrics and Evaluation. 2012. *Financing Global Health 2012: The End of the Golden Age?* Seattle, WA: IHME.

———. 2013. *Global Burden of Disease Study 2010: Results by Cause 1990–2010— Country Level.* Seattle, WA: IHME.

Irwin, Rachel. 2010. "Indonesia, H5N1, and Global Health Diplomacy." *Global Health Governance* 3(2).

Jacobs, Margaret D. 2011. *White Mother to a Dark Race: Settler Colonialism, Mater-*

nalism, and the Removal of Indigenous Children in the American West and Australia, 1880–1940. Lincoln: University of Nebraska Press.

James, Erica Caple. 2010. *Democratic Insecurities: Violence, Trauma, and Intervention in Haiti*. Berkeley: University of California Press.

Jamison, Dean T., et al. 2015. "Global Health 2035: A World Converging within a Generation." *Lancet* 382(9908): 1898–1955.

Janes, Craig R., and O. Chuluundorj. 2004. "Free Markets and Dead Mothers: The Social Ecology of Maternal Mortality in Post-Socialist Mongolia." *Medical Anthropology Quarterly* 18(2): 230–57.

Johnson, Dayo. 2013. "Ondo Tops in Polio Eradication Effort in Nigeria." Vanguard. November 13. http://www.vanguardngr.com/?s=ondo+tops&x=6&y=7.

Jones, David. 2004. *Rationalizing Epidemics: Meanings and Uses of American Indian Mortality since 1600*. Cambridge: Harvard University Press.

Jones, Richard S. 1981. "Alaska Native Claims Settlement Act of 1971 (Public Law 92–203): History and Analysis Together with Subsequent Amendments." Alaskool. June 1. http://www.alaskool.org/projects/ancsa/reports/rsjones1981/ancsa _history71.htm#VII.%20General%20Summary%20of%20the%20Provisions%20of %20the%20Alaska%20Native%20Claims%20Settlement%20Act.

Joseph, May. 1999. "Introduction." In *Nomadic Identities: The Performance of Citizenship*. Minneapolis: University of Minnesota Press.

Justice, Judith. 1986. "Delivering Services to Rural Villages." In *Policies, Plans and People: Culture and Health Development in Nepal*. Berkeley: University of California Press.

Kaler, Amy. 2001. "Many Divorces and Many Spinsters: Marriage as an Invented Tradition in Southern Malawi." *Journal of Family History* 26(4): 529–56.

Kalofonos, Ippolytos. 2014. "'All They Do Is Pray': Community Labour and the Narrowing of 'Care' during Mozambique's HIV Scale-up." *Global Public Health* 9(1–2): 7–24.

Kalt, Joseph P., Eric Henson, Jonathan B. Taylor, Catherine E. A. Curtis, Stephen Cornell, Kenneth W. Grant, Miriam R. Jorgensen, Joseph P. Kalt, and Andrew J. Lee. 2008. *The State of the Native Nations: Conditions under U.S. Policies of Self-Determination*. New York: Oxford University Press.

Kaspin, Deborah. 1996. "A Chewa Cosmology of the Body." *American Ethnologist* 23(3): 561–578.

Katz, Alison. 2008. "New Global Health: A Reversal of Logic, History and Principles." *Social Medicine* 3(1): 1–3.

Kaufert, Patricia, and John D. O'Neil. 1990. "Cooptation and Control: The Reconstruction of Inuit Birth." *Medical Anthropology Quarterly* 4(3): 427–42.

Kawagley, Angayuqaq Oscar. 2006. *A Yupiaq Worldview: A Pathway to Ecology and Spirit*. 2nd ed. Long Grove, IL: Waveland Press.

Kelly, A., and U. Beisel. 2011. "Neglected Malarias: The Frontlines and Back Alleys of Global Health." *BioSocieties* 6(1): 71–87.

Keshavjee, Saalman. 2014. *Blind Spot: How Neoliberalism Infected Global Health*. Berkeley: University of California Press.

Kizer, Kenneth W., and R. Adams Dudley. 2008. "Extreme Makeover: Transformation of the Veterans Health Care System." *Annual Review of Public Health* 30(18.1–18.27): 313–39.

Koch, Erin. 2013. *Free Market Tuberculosis: Managing Epidemics in Postsocialist Georgia.* Nashville: Vanderbilt University Press.

Krause, James S. 1990. "The Relationship between Productivity and Adjustment Following Spinal Cord Injury." *Rehabilitation Counseling Bulletin* 33(3): 188–99.

———. 1992. "Longitudinal Changes in Adjustment after Spinal Cord Injury: A 15-Year Study." *Archives of Physical Medicine and Rehabilitation* 73(6): 564–68.

Krieger, Nancy. 2012. "Methods for the Scientific Study of Discrimination and Health: An Ecosocial Approach." *American Journal of Public Health* 102(5): 936–44.

Kupersmith, Joel, et al. 2007. "Advancing Evidence-based Care for Diabetes: Lessons from the Veterans Health Administration." *Health Affairs* 26(2): w156–w168.

Lakoff, Andrew. 2010. "Two Regimes of Global Health." *Humanity* 1(1): 59–79.

Lambert, Helen. 2006. "Accounting for EBM: Notions of Evidence in Medicine." *Social Science & Medicine* 62: 2633–45.

Lammers, John C., et al. 1996. "Total Quality Management in Hospitals: The Contributions of Commitment, Quality Councils, Teams, Budgets, and Training to Perceived Improvements at Veterans Health Administration Hospitals." *Medical Care* 34(5): 463–78.

Lancet Editorial. 2009. "What Has the Gates Foundation Done for Global Health?" *Lancet* 373: 1577.

Langwick, Stacey. 2012. "The Choreography of Global Subjection: The Traditional Birth Attendant in Contemporary Configurations of World Health." In H. Dilger, A. Kane, and S. Langwick, eds., *Medicine, Mobility and Power in Global Africa: Transnational Health and Healing.* Bloomington: Indiana University Press.

Latour, Bruno. 1987. *Science in Action.* Cambridge: Cambridge University Press.

Lave, Jean. 1988. *Cognition in Practice: Mind, Mathematics and Culture in Everyday Life.* Cambridge: Cambridge University Press.

Lee, Kelley, Susan Erikson, John Calvert, Ann Florini, Ben Hawkins, Chris Holden, Stephen Kcline, Anne Roemer-Mahler, Richard Smith, and Heather Wipfli. 2012. "Corporation Influence on Global Health." Paper presented at Workshop on Corporations and Global Health Diplomacy, Simon Fraser University, September.

Leibow, Edward, Virginia R. Dominquez, Peter Neal Peregrine, Teresa L. McCarty, Mark Nichter, Bonnie Nardy, and Jennifer Leeman. 2013. "Vital Topics Forum: On Evidence and the Public Interest." *American Anthropologist* 115(4): 642–55.

Leins, Stefan. 2011. "Pricing the Revolution: Financial Analysts Respond to the Egyptian Uprising. *Anthropology Today* 27(4): 11–14.

Leite, Iuri C., et al. 2013. "National and Regional Estimates of Disability-Adjusted Life-Years (DALYs) in Brazil, 2008: A Systematic Analysis." *Lancet* 381(s83). http://www.thelancet.com/journals/lancet/article/PIIS0140-6736(13)61337-9/abstract.

Linxwiler, James D. 2007. "The Alaska Native Claims Settlement Act at 35: Delivering on the Promise." 53rd Annual Rocky Mountain Mineral Law Institute, paper 12. http://www.lbblawyers.com/ancsa/ANCSA%20at%2035%20Delivering%20on %20the%20Promise%20Proof%2010-25-07.pdf.

Livingston, Julie. 2012. *Improvising Medicine: An African Oncology Ward in an Emerging Cancer Epidemic*. Durham: Duke University Press.

Loomba, Ania. 2005. *Colonialism/Postcolonialism*. London: Routledge.

Lorway, Robert, and Shamshad Khan. 2014. "Reassembling Epidemiology: Mapping, Monitoring and Making-up People in the Context of HIV Prevention in India." *Social Science and Medicine* 112: 51–62.

Mahal, Ajay, et al. 2013. "What Is a Health Card Worth? A Randomised Controlled Trial of an Outpatient Health Insurance Product in Rural India." *Lancet* 381(S87). http://www.thelancet.com/journals/lancet/article/PIIS0140-6736(13)61341-0 /abstract.

Mahajan, Manjari. 2014. "Ten Years of the Gates Foundation in India." Paper presented at the UCSF GatesKeeping Workshop, Department of Anthropology, History and Social Medicine, University of California, San Francisco, April 18.

Marcus, George. 1995. "Ethnography in/of the World System: The Emergence of Multi-Sited Ethnography." *Annual Review of Anthropology* 24(10): 95–117.

Mathers, Colin, and Ties Boerma. 2010. "Mortality Measurement Matters: Improving Data Collection and Estimation Methods for Child and Adult Mortality." *PLoS Medicine* 7(4): e1000265.

Mattoo, Aaditya, Ileana Cristina Neagu, and Çağlar Özden. 2005. *Brain Waste? Educated Immigrants in the U.S. Labor Market*. World Bank Policy Research Working Paper 3581. Washington, DC: World Bank.

Maurer, Bill. 2013. "The Disunity of Finance: Alternative Practices to Western Finance." In Karin Knorr Cetina and Alex Preda, eds., *The Oxford Handbook of the Sociology of Finance*, 413–30. Oxford: Oxford University Press.

Mayer-Schönberger, Viktor, and Kenneth Cukier. 2014. *Big Data: A Revolution That Will Transform How We Live, Work, and Think*. New York: Eamon Dolan/Mariner Books.

Mbembe, Achille. 2001. *On the Postcolony*. Berkeley: University of California Press.

———. 2003. "Necropolitics." *Public Culture* 15(1): 11–40.

McCarrey, Kristin. 2013. "Alaska Natives: Possessing Inherent Rights to Self-Governance and Self-Governing from Time Immemorial to Present Day." *American Indian Law Journal* 1(2): 437–52.

McCoy, David, Gayatri Kembhavi, Jinesh Patel, and Akish Luintel. 2009. "The Bill & Melinda Gates Foundation's Grant Making Programme for Global Health." *Lancet, Health Policy* 373(May 9): 1645–51.

McCullough, Megan B., Bridget Hahm, and Sarah Ono. 2013. "Observers Observed: Exploring the Practice of Anthropology in the VA." *Annals of Anthropological Practice* 37(2): 5–19.

McGoey, Linsay, Julian Reiss, and Ayo Wahlberg. 2011. "The Global Health Complex." *Biosocieties* 6(1): 1–9.

McQueen, Lynn, Brian S. Bittman, and John G. Demakis. 2004. "Overview of the

Veterans Health Administration (VHA) Quality Enhancement Research Initiative (QUERI)." *Journal of the American Medical Informatics Association* 11(5): 339–43.

Merry, Sally Engle. 2011. "Measuring the World: Indicators, Human Rights, and Global Governance." *Current Anthropology* 52(S3): S83–S95.

Merson, Michael H., Robert E. Black, and Anne J. Mills. 2012. *Global Health: Diseases, Programs, Systems, and Policies*. Burlington, MA: Jones & Bartlett Learning.

Mertens, D. M., and A. T. Wilson. 2012. *Program Evaluation Theory and Practice: A Comprehensive Guide*. New York: Guilford Press.

Metzl, Jonathan M., ed. 2010. *Against Health: How Health Became the New Morality*. New York: New York University Press.

Miles, James A., and John R. Ezzell. 1980. "The Weighted Average Cost of Capital, Perfect Capital Markets and Project Life: A Clarification." *Journal of Financial and Quantitative Analysis* 15(3): 719–730.

Miller, Mark Edwin. 2004. *Forgotten Tribes: Unrecognized Indians and the Federal Acknowledgement Process*. Lincoln: University of Nebraska Press.

Millon, Dian. 2013. *Therapeutic Nations: Healing in the Age of an Indigenous Human Rights*. Tucson: University of Arizona Press.

Ministry of Health and Prevention of Senegal. 2009. *Plan National de Développement Sanitaire 2009–2018*. Dakar: Ministère de la Santé.

Ministry of Health, Republic of Malawi. 2010. *EmONC Needs Assessment Final Report*. Lilongwe: Ministry of Health.

Minn, Pierre. 2011. "'Where They Need Me': The Moral Economy of International Medical Aid in Haiti." PhD diss., McGill University.

Moher, David, Kenneth F. Schulz, and Douglas G. Altman. 2001. "The CONSORT Statement: Revised Recommendation for Improving the Quality of Reports of Parallel Group Randomized Trials." *MBC Medical Research Methodology* 1(2).

Moodie, Megan. 2013. "Microfinance and the Gender of Risk: The Case of Kiva.org." *Signs* 38(2): 279–302.

Mortimer, Duncan, and Leonie Segal. 2008. "Comparing the Incomparable? A Systematic Review of Competing Techniques for Converting Descriptive Measures of Health Status into QALY-Weights." *Medical Decision Making* 28(1): 66–89.

Murray, C. J. L. 1994. "Quantifying the Burden of Disease: The Technical Basis for Disability Adjusted Life Years." *WHO Bulletin OMS* 72: 427–45.

———. 1996. "Rethinking DALYs." In C. J. L. Murray A. and Lopez, eds., *The Global Burden of Disease*. Cambridge: Harvard University Press.

Murray, C. L., and A. D. Lopez. 1994a. "Global and Regional Cause-of-Death Patterns in 1990." *Bulletin of the World Health Organization* 72(3): 447–80.

———. 1994b. "Quantifying Disability: Data, Methods, and Results." *Bulletin of the World Health Organization* 72(3): 481–94.

———. 1996. *The Global Burden of Disease*. Cambridge: Harvard University Press.

———. 2000. "Progress and Directions in Refining the Global Burden of Disease Approach: A Response to Williams." *Health Economics* 9(1): 69–82.

Murray Li, Tania. 2005. "Beyond 'the State' and Failed Schemes." *American Anthropologist* 107(3): 383–94.

————. 2007. *The Will to Improve: Governmentality, Development, and the Practice of Politics.* Durham: Duke University Press.

Nandy, Ashis. 1989. *The Intimate Enemy: Loss and Recovery of Self under Colonialism.* Oxford: Oxford University Press.

National Malaria Control Program of Senegal. 2001. *Plan Strategique Pour Faire Reculer le Paludisme au Senegal.* Dakar: Ministère de la Santé.

————. 2013a. *Note d'Information Supervision Dépots Médicaments du 4 au 22 février 2013.* Dakar: Ministère de la Santé.

————. 2013b.////was a *Revue des Performances À Mi-Parcours du Programme.* Dakar: Ministère de la Santé.

National Population Commission [Nigeria] and ICF Macro. 2009. *Nigeria Demographic and Health Survey 2008.* Abuja, Nigeria: NPC and ICF Macro.

National Statistical Office and ICF Macro. 2011. *Malawi Demographic and Health Survey 2010.* Calverton, MD: NSO and ICF Macro.

Navarro, Vicente. 1978. *Medicine under Capitalism.* Ann Arbor: University of Michigan Press.

Nguyen, Vinh-Kim. 2010. *The Republic of Therapy: Triage and Sovereignty in West Africa's Time of AIDS.* Durham: Duke University Press.

Nichter, Mark. 2008. *Global Health: Why Cultural Perceptions, Social Representations and Biopolitics Matter.* Tucson: University of Arizona Press.

————. 2013. "The Rise and Transformation of Evidence-Based Medicine." In Edward Leibow et al. *American Anthropologist* 115(4): 647–49.

Oliver, Adam. 2007. "The Veterans Health Administration: An American Success Story?" *Milbank Quarterly* 85(1): 5–35.

Ong, Aihwa. 2006. *Neoliberalism as Exception: Mutations in Citizenship and Sovereignty.* Durham: Duke University Press.

Osseo-Asare, Abena. 2014. *Bitter Roots: The Search for Healing Plants in Africa.* Chicago: University of Chicago Press.

Ottomanelli, Lisa, et al. 2012. "Effectiveness of Supported Employment for Veterans with Spinal Cord Injuries: Results from a Randomized Multisite Study." *Archives of Physical Medicine and Rehabilitation:* 740–47.

Outcome Mapping Learning Community. N.d. Accessed July 1, 2014.

Packard, Randall M. 1989. *White Plague, Black Labor: Tuberculosis and the Political Economy of Health and Disease in South Africa.* Berkeley: University of California Press.

————. 1997a. "Malaria Dreams: Postwar Visions of Health and Development in the Third World." *Medical Anthropology* 17(3): 279–96.

————. 1997b. "Visions of Postwar Health and Development and Their Impact on Public Health Intervention in the Developing World." In F. Cooper and R. Packard, eds., *International Development and the Social Sciences,* 93–115. Berkeley: University of California Press.

————. 2011. *The Making of a Tropical Disease: A Short History of Malaria.* Baltimore: Johns Hopkins University Press.

Palmer, Steven. 2010. *Launching Global Heath: The Caribbean Odyssey of the Rockefeller Foundation*. Ann Arbor: University of Michigan Press.

Pandolfi, Mariella, and Didier Fassin. 2007. *Contemporary States of Emergency*. Boston: MIT Press.

Parker, Melissa, and Tim Allen. 2014. "De-Politicizing Parasites: Reflections on Attempts to Control Neglected Tropical Diseases." *Medical Anthropology* 33(3): 223–39.

Partnering for Global Health Forum. 2011. "Accounting for Global Health: Understanding Funding Opportunities." Panel session at Partnering for Global Health Forum, June 27, Washington, DC. Accessed November 2, 2013. http://www3.bio.org/pgh/program/accounting-for-global-health/.

PATH. 2010. *Staying the Course? Malaria Research and Development in a Time of Economic Uncertainty*. Seattle: PATH.

Peterman, Amber, et al. 2013. "Income Shocks and Material Health: Evidence from a Large-Scale Randomised Cash Transfer Experiment in Zambia." *Lancet* 381(S109). http://www.thelancet.com/journals/lancet/article/PIIS0140-6736(13)61363-X/abstract.

Peterson, Kristin. 2014. *Speculative Markets: Drug Circuits and Derivative Life in Nigeria*. Durham: Duke University Press.

Petryna, Adriana. 2009. *When Experiments Travel: Clinical Trials and the Global Search for Human Subjects*. Princeton: Princeton University Press.

Pfeiffer, James. 2004. "Condom Social Marketing, Pentecostalism, and Structural Adjustment in Mozambique: A Clash of AIDS Prevention Messages." *Medical Anthropology Quarterly* 18(1): 77–103.

Pfeiffer, James, and Rachel Chapman. 2010. "Anthropological Perspectives on Structural Adjustment and Public Health." *Annual Review of Anthropology* 39: 149–65.

Piatote, Beth. 2013. *Domestic Subjects: Gender, Citizenship, and Law in Native American Literature*. New Haven: Yale University Press.

Pigg, Stacy Leigh. 1996. "The Credible and the Credulous: The Question of 'Villagers' Beliefs' in Nepal." *Cultural Anthropology* 11(2): 160–201.

———. 1997. "Authority in Translation: Finding, Knowing, Naming, and Training 'Traditional Birth Attendants' in Nepal." In R. Davis-Floyd and C. F. Sargent, eds., *Childbirth and Authoritative Knowledge: Cross-Cultural Perspectives*. Berkeley: University of California Press.

———. 2013. "On Sitting and Doing: Ethnography as action in global health" *Social Science and Medicine* 99:C: 127–34.

Piketty, Thomas. 2014. *Capital in the Twenty-First Century*. Trans. Arthur Goldhammer. Cambridge: Belknap Press of Harvard University Press.

Pisani, Elizabeth. 2009. *The Wisdom of Whores: Bureaucrats, Brothels and the Business of AIDS*. New York: Norton.

Porter, Theodore M. 1986. *The Rise of Statistical Thinking 1820–1900*. Princeton: Princeton University Press.

———. 1992. "Quantification and the Accounting Ideal in Science." *Social Studies of Science* 22(4): 633–51.

————. 1995. *Trust in Numbers: The Pursuit of Objectivity in Science and Public Life.* Princeton: Princeton University Press.

Povinelli, Elizabeth. 2006. *The Empire of Love: Toward a Theory of Intimacy, Genealogy, and Carnality.* Durham: Duke University Press.

Prakash, Gyan. 1999. *Another Reason: Science and the Imagination of Modern India.* Princeton: Princeton University Press.

Rajan, Kaushik Sunder. 2006. *Biocapital: The Constitution of Postgenomic Life.* Durham: Duke University Press.

————. 2012. "Pharmaceutical Crises and Questions of Value: Terrains and Logics of Global Therapeutic Politics." *South Atlantic Quarterly* 111(2): 321–46.

Rapkin, Bruce D., and Edison J. Trickett. 2005. "Comprehensive Dynamic Trial Designs for Behavioral Prevention Research with Communities: Overcoming Inadequacies of the Randomized Controlled Trial Paradigm." In Edison J. Trickett and Willo Pequegnat, eds., *Community Interventions and AIDS,* 249. Oxford: Oxford University Press.

Redfield, Peter. 2006. "A Less Modest Witness: Collective Advocacy and Motivated Truth in a Medical Humanitarian Movement." *American Ethnologist* 33(1): 3–26.

————. 2013. *Life in Crisis: The Ethical Journey of Doctors without Borders.* Berkeley: University of California Press.

Rees, Tobias. (n.d.) *Today, What Is Humanity? An Anthropological Study of Global Health.*

————. 2014. "Humanity/Plan; Or, on the 'Stateless' Today (Also Being an Anthropology of Global Health)." *Cultural Anthropology.*

Reubi, David. 2013. "Health Economists, Tobacco Control and International Development: On the Economization of Global Health beyond Neoliberal Structural Adjustment Policies." *BioSocieties* (2013): 8, 205–28.

Reynolds Whyte, Susan. 2014. *Second Chances: Surviving AIDS in Uganda.* Durham: Duke University Press.

Roll Back Malaria Partnership. 2010. *Roll Back Malaria Progress and Impact Series: Malaria Funding and Resource Utilization. The First Decade of Roll Back Malaria.* UNICEF, WHO, PATH.

Rose Hunt, Nancy. 1999. *A Colonial Lexicon: Of Birth Ritual, Medicalization, and Mobility in the Congo.* Durham: Duke University Press.

Roy, Ananya. 2010. *Poverty Capital.* Berkeley: University of California Press.

————. 2012. "Ethical Subjects: Market Rule in an Age of Poverty." *Public Culture* 24(1 66): 105–8. doi:10.1215/08992363–1443574.

Roy, Arundhati. 2011. *Public Power in the Age of Empire.* New York: Seven Stories Press.

Saez, Emmanuel. 2013. "Striking It Richer: The Evolution of Top Incomes in the United States." Updated version. *Pathways Magazine,* Stanford Center for the Study of Poverty and Inequality (Winter 2008): 6–7. Accessed November 3, 2013. http://eml.berkeley.edu//~saez/saez-UStopincomes-2013.pdf.

Sane, Idrissa. 2013. Sécurité de la santé: Le Sutsas/Sas lève le mot d'ordre de rétention des données sanitaires. Le Soleil, March 3.

Sangaramoorthy, Thurka. 2012. "Treating the Numbers: HIV/AIDS Surveillance Subjectivity and Risk." *Medical Anthropology* 31(4): 292–309.

Sangaramoorthy, Thurka, and Adia Benton. 2012. "Introduction: Enumeration, Identity, and Health." *Medical Anthropology* 31: 287–91.

Saul, Jason. 2014. "Cracking the Code on Social Impact." Video. Skoll World Forum, April 9. Accessed January 14, 2015. http://skollworldforum.org/session/skoll-world-forum-2014/seminars/cracking-code-social-impact/?play=cracking-code-social-impact#videos.

Schlander, Michael. 2010. "Measures of Efficiency in Healthcare: QALMs about QALYs?" *Zeitschrift für Evidenz, Fortbildung und Qualität im Gesundheitswesen* 104(3): 214–26.

Schoffeleers, Matthew. 2000. "The Story of a Scapegoat King in Rural Malawi." In R. van Dijk, R. Reis, and M. Spierenburg, eds., *The Quest for Fruition through Ngoma: Political Aspects of Healing in Southern Africa*, 99–116. Oxford: James Currey.

Schuller, Mark. 2012. *Killing With Kindness?: Haiti, International Aid and NGOs*. New Brunswick: Rutgers University Press.

Schulz, Kenneth F., et al. 2010. "CONSORT 2010 Statement: Updated Guidelines for Reporting Parallel Group Randomized Trials." *Annals of Internal Medicine* 152(11): 1–7.

Scott, James. 1999. *Seeing Like a State: How Certain Schemes to Improve the Human Condition Have Failed*. New Haven: Yale University Press.

Secretariat du Comité Central du PIT. 2011. "L'Atteinte des OMD par notre pays passe par la résolution de la crise sociale dans le secteur de la santé!" Le Blog de Nioxor Tine. April 14. http://www.nioxor.com/search/L%E2%80%99Atteinte%20des%20OMD%20par%20onotre%20pays%20passe%20par%201a%20r%C3%A9solution%20de%201a%20crise%20sociale%20dans%201e%20secteur%20de%201a%20sant%C3%A9/.

Serajuddin, Umar, Nobuo Yoshida, and Hiroki Eamatsu. 2015. "Much of the World Is Deprived of Poverty Data. Let's Fix This." Let's Talk Development: A Blog Hosted by the World Bank's Chief Economist. April 30.

Sexton, Sarah. 2003. "GATS, Privatisation and Health." Corner House. May 11. Accessed June 26, 2014. http://www.thecornerhouse.org.uk/resource/gats-privatisation-and-health.

Shah, Sonia. 2010. *The Fever: How Malaria Has Ruled Mankind for 500,000 Years*. New York: Sarah Crichton Books.

Shore, Cris, and Susan Wright. 2015. "Governing by Numbers: Audit Culture, Rankings and the New World Order." *Social Anthropology* 23(1): 22–28.

Silverstein, Brian. 2014. "Statistics, Reform, and Regimes of Expertise in Turkey." *Turkish Studies* 15(4): 638–54.

Simpson, Audra. 2014. *Mohawk Interruptus: Political Life across the Borders of Settler States*. Durham: Duke University Press.

Singogo, E., et al. 2013. "Village Registers for Vital Registration in Malawi." *Tropical Medicine and International Health* 18(8): 1021–24.

Skolnick, Richard. 2012. *Global Health 101: Second Edition*. Burlington, MA: Jones & Bartlett Learning.

Smith, Stephanie. 2010. "Doubling of Maternal Deaths in U.S. 'Scandalous,' Rights Group Says." CNN news release, March 12.

Smith-Morris, Carolyn, et al. 2013. "Narrating a Return to Work after Spinal Cord Injury." In N. Warren and L. Manderson, eds., *Reframing Disability and Quality of Life: A Global Perspective*, 145–62. Dordrecht: Springer.

Smith-Morris, Carolyn, Gilberto Lopez, Lisa Ottomanelli, Lance Goetz, and Kimberly Dixon-Lawson. 2014. "Ethnography, Fidelity and the Evidence Anthropology Adds: Supplementing the Fidelity Process in a Clinical Trial of Supported Employment." *Medical Anthropology Quarterly* 28(2): 141–61.

Smith-Morris, Carolyn, ed. 2015. *Diagnostic Controversy: Cultural Perspectives on Competing Knowledge in Healthcare*. New York: Routledge.

Sobo, Elisa J. 2009. *Culture and Meaning in Health Services Research: A Practical Field Guide*. Walnut Creek, CA: Left Coast Press.

Staples, Amy L. S. 2006. *The Birth of Development: How the World Bank, Food and Agriculture Organization, and World Health Organization Have Changed the World (1945–1965)*. Kent, OH: Kent State University Press.

Stepan, Nancy Leys. 2011. *Eradication: Ridding the World of Diseases Forever?* Ithaca: Cornell University Press.

Stetler, Cheryl B., Brian S. Mittman, and Joseph Francis. 2008. "Overview of the VA Quality Enhancement Research Initiative." *Implementation Science* 3: 8.

Stevenson, Lisa. 2012. "The Psychic Life of Biopolitics: Survival, Cooperation, and Inuit Community." *American Ethnologist* 39(3): 592–613.

―――. 2014. *Life beside Itself: Imagining Care in the Canadian Arctic*. Berkeley: University of California Press.

Storeng, Katerini T., and Dominique P. Behague. 2014. "'Playing the Numbers Game': Evidence-based Advocacy and the Technocratic Narrowing of the Safe Motherhood Initiative." *Medical Anthropology* 28(2): 260–79.

Strathern, Marilyn. 2005. "Robust Knowledge and Fragile Futures." In Aihwa Ong and Stephen J. Collier, eds., *Global Assemblages: Technology, Politics, and Ethics as Anthropological Problems*. Malden, MA: Blackwell.

Stuckler, David, Sanjay Basu, and Martin McKee. 2011. "Global Health Philanthropy and Institutional Relationships: How Should Conflicts of Interest Be Addressed?" *PLoS Medicine* 8(4).

Sullivan, Paul. 2014. "Investing to Make a Difference Is Gaining Ground." *New York Times*, September 5.

Sunder Rajan, Kaushik. 2006. *Biocapital: The Constitution of Postgenomic Life*. Durham: Duke University Press.

Swinburn, Boyd A., Gary Sacks, Kevin D. Hall, Klim McPherson, Diane T. Finegood, Marjory L. Moodie, and Steven L. Gortmaker. 2011. "The Global Obesity Pandemic: Shaped by Global Drivers and Local Environments." *Lancet* 378(9793): 804–14.

Taussig, Michael T. 1980. "Reification and the Consciousness of the Patient." *Social Science & Medicine* 14(11): 3–13.

Thaddeus, Sereen, and Deborah Maine. 1994. "Too Far to Walk: Maternal Mortality in Context." *Social Science & Medicine* 38(8): 1091–110.

Tesfai, Casie, Ruwan Ratnayake, and Mark Myatt. 2013. "Measuring Local Determinants of Acute Malnutrition in Chad: A Case-Control Study." *Lancet* 381(S144). http://www.thelancet.com/journals/lancet/article/PIIS0140-6736(13)61398-7/abstract.

Thiam, Mballo Dia. 2012. "Rapport Moral du Secrétaire Général National." 8ème Congrès Ordinaire de SUTSAS et UNSAS. December 21–23. King Fahd Palace Ex Méridien Président, Dakar, Senegal.

———. 2013. "Inégalités et Territorialités: Etat des lieux en matière d'inégalités sociales de santé et écarts dans la distribution des ressources humaines et matériels." Colloque francophone international sur les inégalités sociales de santé en Afrique. May 21–23. Hôtel des Almadies, Dakar, Senegal.

Tilley, Helen. 2011. *Africa as a Living Laboratory: Empire, Development and the Problem of Scientific Knowledge, 1870–1950*. Chicago: University of Chicago Press.

Timmermans, Stefan. 2015. "Trust in Standards: Transitioning Clinical Exome Sequencing from Bench to Bedside." *Social Studies of Science* 45(1): 77–99.

Timmermans, Stefan, and Marc Berg. 2003. *The Gold Standard: The Challenge of Evidence Based Medicine*. Philadelphia: Temple University Press.

Tousignant, Noemi. 2013. "The Qualities of Citizenship: Private Pharmacists and the State in Senegal after Independence and Alternance." In Ruth J. Prince and Rebecca Marsland, eds., *The Making and Unmaking of Public Health in Africa*. Athens: Ohio University Press.

Trieschmann, R. B. 1980. "The Psychological, Social, and Vocational Adjustment to Spinal Cord Injury." *Annual Review of Rehabilitation* 1: 304–18.

Tsing, Anna. 2012. "On Nonscalability: The Living World Is Not Amenable to Precision-Nested Scales." *Common Knowledge* 18(3): 505–24.

United Nations Children's Rights and Emergency Relief Organization. 2007. *The State of the World's Children 2008: Child Survival*. New York: UNICEF.

Vandenbroucke, Jan P. 2008. "Observational Research, Randomised Trials, and Two Views of Medical Science." *PLoS Medicine* 5(3): 0339–43.

Van Hollen, Cecilia. 2013. *Birth in the Age of AIDS: Women, Reproduction, and HIV/AIDS in India*. Stanford: Stanford University Press.

Vaughan, Megan. 2001. *Curing Their Ills: Colonial Power and African Illness*. Stanford: Stanford University Press.

Verran, Helen. 2001. *Science and an African Logic*. Chicago: University of Chicago Press.

Wahlberg, Ayo, and Nikolas Rose. 2015. "The Governmentalization of Living: Calculating Global Health." *Economy and Society* 44(1): 60–90.

Wainwright, Babette. 2001. "Do Something for Your Soul: Go to Haiti." In Edwidge Danticat, ed., *The Butterfly's Way: Voices from the Haitian Dyaspora in the United States*, 204–8. New York: Soho Press.

Waitzkin, Howard. 2011. *Medicine and Public Health at the End of Empire*. Boulder, CO: Paradigm.

Watts, Michael. 1994. "Development II: The Privatization of Everything?" *Progress in Human Geography* 18: 371–84.

Weisz, George. 2005. "From Clinical Counting to Evidence-Based Medicine." In G. Weisz, Gérard Jorland, and Annick Opinel, eds., *Body Counts: Medical Quantification in Historical and Sociological Perspectives / Perspectives historiques et sociologiques sur la quantification médicale*. Montreal: McGill-Queens University Press.

Wendland, Claire. 2010. *A Heart for the Work: Journeys through an African Medical School*. Chicago: University of Chicago Press.

Westgren, N., and R. Levi. 1998. "Quality of Life and Traumatic Spinal Cord Injury." *Archives of Physical Medicine and Rehabilitation* 79(11): 1433–39.

Whyte, Susan Reynolds. 2011. "Writing Knowledge and Acknowledgement: Possibilities in Medical Research." In P. Wenzel Geissler and Catherine Molyneux, eds., *Evidence, Ethos and Experiment: The Anthropology and History of Medical Research in Africa*. Oxford: Berghahn Books.

Wilkinson, Charles. 2005. *Blood Struggle: The Rise of Modern Indian Nations*. New York: Norton.

Williams, Alan. 1999. "Calculating the Global Burden of Disease: Time for a Strategic Reappraisal?" *Health Economics* 8: 1–8.

Williams, Ben A. 2010. "Perils of Evidence-based Medicine." *Perspectives in Biology and Medicine* 53(1): 106–20.

Wilmoth, John R., et al. 2012. "A New Method for Deriving Global Estimates of Maternal Mortality." *Statistics, Politics, and Policy* 3(2): article 3.

World Bank. 2014. "Toward Universal Health Coverage by 2030." April 11. Accessed June 18, 2014. http://live.worldbank.org/toward-universal-health-coverage-2030.

World Health Organization. 2006. *Working Together for Health: The World Health Report 2006*.

———. 2010. "Trends in Maternal Mortality: 1990 to 2008. WHO, UNICEF, UNFPA and The World Bank Estimates." http://www.who.int/whr/2006/en/.

Wubneh, M. 2003. "Building Capacity in Africa: The Impact of Institutional, Policy and Resource Factors." *African Development Review* 15(2/3): 165–98.

Yamey, Gavin. 2011. "Cambodia's Doomed PREP Trial: What Happened Next?" PLoS Blogs. April 14. Accessed June 9, 2014. http://blogs.plos.org/speakingofmedicine /2011/04/14/cambodia%E2%80%99s-doomed-prep-trial-what-happened-next/.

Yerxa, A. Elizabeth J., and Susan Baum. 1986. "Engagement in Daily Occupations and Life Satisfaction among People with Spinal Cord Injuries." *Occupational Therapy Journal of Research* 6(5): 271–83.

CONTRIBUTORS

VINCANNE ADAMS is a professor of medical anthropology in the Department of Anthropology, History and Social Medicine at University of California, San Francisco. Her most recent book is *Markets of Sorrow, Labors of Faith: New Orleans in the Wake of Katrina* (Duke University Press, 2013).

SUSAN L. ERIKSON is an associate professor in the Faculty of Health Sciences and faculty affiliate in the Department of Sociology and Anthropology at Simon Fraser University in Vancouver, British Columbia. She conducts ethnographic research on global health futures and the political economy of biomedicine. Her work has been published in *The Lancet, Foreign Affairs, BMJ series, Community Development, Social Science and Medicine, Medical Anthropology,* and *Global Public Health*.

MOLLY HALES is an MD/PhD candidate in the Medical Scientist Training Program at the University of California, San Francisco, currently completing her PhD in medical anthropology at the University of California, San Francisco and Berkeley, and her MD at the University of California, San Francisco. She has conducted research on gender and HIV in South Africa and the use of metrics in Native American health.

PIERRE MINN is an assistant professor in the Department of Anthropology at the Univ·ersité de Montréal. He has conducted ethnographic research on international medical aid in Haiti and global health education in North

American universities. His current research examines the practices and stakes of knowledge production in Haiti.

ADEOLA ONI-ORISAN is a PhD candidate in the Joint University of California, San Francisco–University of California, Berkeley Program in medical anthropology and an MD candidate at Harvard Medical School. Her current research focuses on development, religion, and reproductive health in Nigeria.

CAROLYN SMITH-MORRIS is an associate professor and the director of the Health and Society Program in the Department of Anthropology at Southern Methodist University. She is the editor of *Diagnostic Controversy: Cultural Perspectives on Competing Knowledge in Healthcare* (2015) and coeditor with Lenore Manderson of *Chronic Conditions, Fluid States: Chronicity and the Anthropology of Illness* (2010).

MARLEE TICHENOR is a PhD candidate from the Joint Medical Anthropology Program at the University of California, Berkeley, and the University of California, San Francisco. Her doctoral thesis, "Malarial Proximities: Senegal, the Pursuit of Evidence, and the Silver Revolver Approach to Global Health," investigates the local health fight against malaria in Senegal and its points of convergence and contention with global malaria governance.

LILY WALKOVER is a PhD candidate in medical sociology in the Department of Social and Behavioral Sciences at the University of California, San Francisco. She has a background in global public health, HIV, and health education.

CLAIRE L. WENDLAND is an associate professor in the Departments of Anthropology, Obstetrics and Gynecology, and Medical History and Bioethics at the University of Wisconsin, Madison. She is the author of *A Heart for the Work: Journeys through an African Medical School* (2010). Her current research focuses on medical expertise in African settings and explanations for maternal death in Malawi.

INDEX

labor unions, 105, 110–14, 120–22, 123n4
Lancet, 24, 37
life satisfaction, 192
local knowledge: in behavioral health programs, 129; compromised by health metrics, 137; definition and use, 143
logarithmic transformation, 72, 81n19

malaria, 105–10, 115–24
Malawi, 59–60, 62–66, 69, 71, 74–76
maternal and child health, 89, 94
maternal death: defined, 80n12; global, 57–59; and HIV/AIDS, 57, 68, 80n16; in Malawi, 59–60, 63–66, 74–76; and maternal mortality, 83, 87, 90, 93; rate, 83, 92; in the United States, 61
maternal mortality ratio: in Africa, 66; defined, 65; global, 58, 66; in Equatorial Guinea, 81n18; and health infrastructure, 62–63; in Iceland, 69, 81n17; in Malawi, 62, 65, 69, 71, 76; political implications, 62, 78; in the United States, 70
maturation of the Health Services Research Field, 203
metrics, and epistemology, 73; influence on health policy, 61–62, 71, 74, 77, 79nn3–4; metric quantification over case-specific quality, 188; and productivity, 85; unembellished, 187
Millenium Development Goals (MDG), 23, 86, 89, 92, 106, 107, 114, 230; and Goal Five, 57, 59–60, 62
multidisciplinarity, 195

narrative, 191, 195, 200
National Science Foundation (NSF), 38
native sovereignty, 135–36; and federal recognition, 128; and Yup'ik behavioral health programs, 130
Nigeria Demographic and Health Survey (NDHS), 86–87
Nigerian Governor's Immunization Leadership Challenge, 87–89
non-governmental Organization (NGO), 47, 88, 92, 164–66, 174–75, 206
numbers, 83, 97, 98; and accountability, 9–10; as common language, 61; as fe-

tishes, 75; as neutral, 61; as political instruments, 84–85, 89–90, 92, 99; and politics, 100; production of, 90, 93, 94

obfuscations, 203
objectivity, 19–20
Office of Research and Development, 191, 207
optimal modes of care, 188
outcome mapping, 172–73
outcomes, 187–89, 191, 193, 194, 196, 200, 204, 205, 207; and outcome-driven context, 188

Pan American Health Organization (PAHO), 3
Partners In Health (PIH), 229
pharmaceuticals, 31; and pharmacovigilance, 113
Pogge, Thomas, 151–52
polio, 87; eradication, 88
politics, 91–92, 94, 96, 98, 100; and economy of health, 85; and efficacy, 85, 99; and global health aid, 89; and goals, 84–85, 93, 98; and health aims, 205; and metrics productivity, 85; numbers and, 100; political capital, 91; and politicization, 204
postcolonial, definition, 126; as denial of legitimacy, 140; and development, 25; and nation state, 3; structures of debt and finance, 131–32
Poverty Action Lab, 33, 52n28
Principle of the Model, 195
PubMed-indexed, 193, 194
purchasing power parity, 80n13

QALY, 26–27, 34
qualitative research, 188, 190, 191, 193, 195, 200, 204–7; and evidence, 195, 200; and publication conventions, 198; and reliability, 194; and replicability, 194, 200
Quality Assurance, 188; and improvement, 188, 189, 202; of life; 191, 192
Quality Enhancement Research Initiative (QUERI), 189, 191, 193, 202, 203, 206